BIOETHICS IN THE 21st CENTURY

Edited by **Abraham Rudnick**

Bioethics in the 21st Century
Edited by Abraham Rudnick

Published by InTech

Janeza Trdine 9, 51000 Rijeka, Croatia

Publishing Process Manager Sandra Bakic

Technical Editor Teodora Smiljanic

Cover Designer InTech Design Team

Additional hard copies can be obtained from orders@intechopen.com

Bioethics in the 21st Century, Edited by Abraham Rudnick
p. cm.
ISBN 978-953-307-270-8

For EU product safety concerns:
IN TECH d.o.o., Prolaz Marije Krucifikse Kozulić 3, 51000 Rijeka, Croatia,
info@intechopen.com or visit our website at intechopen.com.

Meet the editor

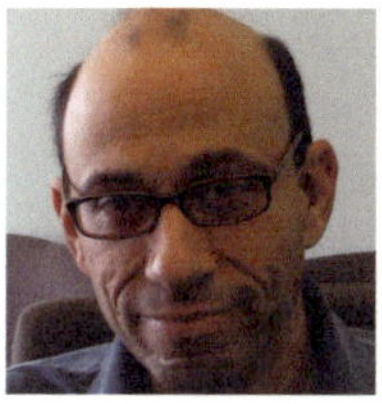

Dr. Abraham (Rami) Rudnick, BMedSc, MD, MPsych, PhD, CPRP, FRCPC, is an Associate Professor, Departments of Psychiatry and Philosophy, The University of Western Ontario, Canada. His academic interests center on the ethics, epistemology and metaphysics of health care and related research and on interventions – particularly psychosocial – for people with serious mental illness such as schizophrenia. He has published about dialogue in bioethics, capacity to make decisions about treatment, and health as self-organization, among other topics. Some of his recent academic work challenges widely accepted notions such as (medical) invasiveness and standard principles of bioethics. He is the founder and Head of the Canadian Unit of the International Network of the UNESCO Chair in Bioethics (Haifa), which focuses on development, evaluation and dissemination of bioethics education. His work is motivated by the belief that philosophical inquiry is beneficial for health care practice, research, education and administration.

Contents

1

Introduction to Bioethics in the 21st Century

Abraham Rudnick* and Kyoko Wada
Departments of Psychiatry and Philosophy and Faculty of Health Sciences, The University of Western Ontario Canada

1. Introduction

Health care is developing rapidly. So are its correlates, such as health care technology, research, education, administration, communication, and more. Such change requires ethical deliberation, as change that is not ethically guided poses unnecessary risks. This may be particularly true in relation to health care, which impacts some of the most central domains of human life. Bioethics addresses issues of health care ethics. It consists of approaches that attempt to resolve moral conflicts, viewed as conflicts among moral values that may each be acceptable in some circumstances but that require prioritizing when combined with other moral values in particular circumstances. Such approaches include the application of theories such as consequentialism, which refers to outcomes (such as happiness); deontology, which refers to duties or intentions (such as the obligation not to lie); virtue ethics, which refers to character features (such as honesty); principlism, which refers to the four principles of upholding autonomy (self-determination), beneficence (best interests), non-maleficence (least harm), and justice (as fairness, for example); and more (Beauchamp & Childress, 2009; Rudnick, 2001; Rudnick, 2002).

Bioethics ranges across many areas and its scope is still broadening. Some of its emerging areas address organizational bioethics, global bioethics, and much more. This book focuses on a sample of emerging as well as more established areas of bioethics. The chapters were selected according to various considerations, such as interest of authors. Yet in spite of not being exhaustive, this book illustrates the range and impact of bioethics in the 21st century. As part of that, some of the chapters go beyond fact and theory into some speculation (the chapters with more speculative topics can be found near the end of this book). We think this is necessary for bioethics to be constructive, recognizing that speculation must be checked by common sense as well as by known fact and theory. Indeed this is how much of bioethics proceeds (Rudnick 2007).

There are areas of bioethics that are not covered in this book, such as neuroethics, enhancement ethics, ethics of genetics, and more. We cannot touch on most of them here. Still, we would like to highlight neuroethics as a likely paradigm of an emerging area in bioethics. Neuroethics can be defined in part as the ethics of neuroscience (http://en.wikipedia.org/wiki/Neuroethics). More specifically, it can be viewed in part as

---

* arudnic2@uwo.ca

the ethics of brain assessment and manipulation with advanced technology, such as transcranial magnetic stimulation (TMS) and (electric) deep brain stimulation (DBS); these technologies may induce important intended and unintended brain changes. Such brain assessment and manipulation has implications for personal identity, self-determination, social influence on health care, and more. Much if not all of this is not new, yet in neuroethics it is perhaps more prominent than elsewhere and may require new approaches and solutions. Such emerging bioethics may contribute to ethics more generally, be it by generating new problems and/or by generating new solutions to old problems that emerging and established health care practices and related technologies raise in variant forms. We hope this book will be part of this contribution in the areas that it addresses and beyond. The editor (first author of this introductory chapter), would like to point out that due to the publishing process of the book, he cannot take full responsibility for the substance and style of this book. Such open access publication is a fairly new part of bioethics in the 21st century, and as such the book exemplifies an aspect of its subject matter.

2. Overview of chapters

In chapter 2, Beca and Astete discuss the issue of decision-making in relation to patients who have no plausible prospect of recovery. They focus on examples where life support may no longer be meaningful but rather may prolong the suffering of the patient and the family members. As is illustrated in one of the four examples presented, some family members may hold an unrealistic hope for recovery, no matter what the circumstances may be. Also, it can be stressful for healthcare professionals to withdraw or limit any kind of life prolonging procedures. The authors apply the principlist approach to grapple with the difficulties involved in end-of-life decision-making (although distributive justice as related to resource allocation can be viewed as part of principlism, it is not discussed in this chapter). They argue that in terms of autonomy, the patient's values must be respected; however, the patient may not be fully capable of making his or her own decisions, and the substitute decision maker (SDM) may not necessarily know the patient's values. Considering a variety of difficulties involved in this decision-making process, the authors argue for shared decision-making by several agents, such as healthcare professionals and ethics representatives, in addition to the patient and his or her SDM. Shared decision-making pursues a balance of benefits and burdens, which may secure the patient's best interests. Such an approach may appear to have an emphasis on beneficence more than on autonomy. But, as is the bioethical standard now, the authors' argumentation portrays beneficence as what is good for the patient based on his or her values (when known). Hence, autonomy trumps, unless neither the past nor the present values of the patient can be known (in which case, autonomy may be irrelevant).

In chapter 3, Russell argues that ethical considerations involved in mental health and addiction settings do not stand alone but co-exist with clinical, legal, organizational and other considerations. Seven examples involving ethical complexities are presented in the beginning to illustrate issues arising from the care of those with mental illnesses and/or addictions; these issues are addressed later in the chapter. These examples are not as dramatic as may be often displayed to the general public through media, but are rich with issues encountered in daily healthcare practice, education and management. In these examples, we encounter patients as well as a wide range of other agents, such as their family members, a landlord, a judge, a clinical director of an organization, and others who are related to the patient through their mental health and addiction problems or otherwise. Following discussion of being humane, being a person, being a community member, and being a care provider, all of which comprise ethical considerations, the author proceeds to discuss why other factors matter ethically. Among these are science, technology and clinical factors, law and regulations, organizational contexts, and systemic factors, such as stigma and discrimination, the social determinants of health and the health care system.

In chapter 4, Putoto and Pegoraro discuss resource allocation, which is among the most important and pressing issues in healthcare today, both in developed and in developing countries. As resources are limited, we must make a difficult choice to achieve the goal of efficient and effective healthcare. Rationing, defined by the authors as "the distribution of resources between programmes and persons in competition", needs to be done explicitly and at various levels, i.e. from policy making to individual care. However, as the authors argue, we are far from reaching a consensus in terms of who decides and what the guiding strategies should be. Several approaches to rationing are possible. Experiences of a few jurisdictions are classified into three models. The first model, which is employed in Oregon (United States), explicitly identifies a list of treatments to be publicly funded. The second model, which is employed in the Netherlands and Sweden, adopts some principles to identify available treatments or priorities in the provision of healthcare. The third model, which is employed in New Zealand and Great Britain, relies on specific guidelines regarding treatments, and the rationing is done at the local and individual levels. However, as the authors indicate, none of these models are without problems, and no matter what model we use, there will always be ambiguities. More discussion on rationing is required regarding resource allocation.

In chapter 5, Ravez analyzes ethical criticism of employing procreation technologies. He also presents his proposal regarding the issues arising from these new technologies for couples who want to have a bio-child. From his review of literature, particularly that written in French, he classifies ethical criticism of medically assisted procreation (MAP) into three types: medicalization of procreation, the dissociation of biological and social filiation, and the controversial status of the embryo. Ravez recognizes that these criticisms are not without counter arguments and may not necessarily be limited to MAP. Moreover, these criticisms may dismiss the effectiveness of these new technologies which may enable a couple to satisfy their legitimate desire to have a bio-child. He claims that we should not deny the suffering of sterile couples and proposes a framework to address the ethical issues involved in MAP. According to him, first, we must listen to couples who are suffering from sterility and discern how their sterility may or may not relate to their suffering. Second, we must respect the complexity of life. Having a child cannot be reduced to a simple biological phenomenon but involves various other important elements, such as family relationships and psychological aspects. Third, these new technologies should be understood as a means to help the sterile couple have children (rather than preselect or enhance their children, for example). The framework urges us to acknowledge the suffering of those with sterility; concomitantly, it provides certain requirements to ethically regulate MAP.

In chapter 6, Zahedi-Anaraki and Larijani discuss ethical issues related to stem cell research and its potential clinical applications. As stem cells have the capacity to differentiate into a variety of cells which may be employed for therapeutic purposes, research has held much hope and enthusiasm for their positive contribution to the treatment of currently incurable illnesses. At the same time, such research, particularly that employing embryonic stem cells, has been criticized as it involves ethical challenges, some of which are related to personhood and human dignity. The chapter begins with definitions and characteristics of several types of stem cells. The ethical issues discussed in this chapter include human dignity in relation to the instrumentalization and destruction of human embryos, safety concerns in clinical applications of stem cell use, informed consent for conducting procedures involving stem cells, slippery slope arguments regarding the creation and use of human embryos, resource allocation and commercialization of stem cell therapies. In addition, the authors refer to legislation and guidelines concerning stem cell research by national and international regulatory bodies as well as positions expressed by religious authorities, such as in Christianity, Judaism and Islam. The authors conclude by indicating the need for research on alternatives to embryonic stem cells, such as induced pluripotent stem cells, for realistic regulations in relation to stem cell research, for control of commercialism, and for more engagement of the public.

In chapter 7, Nie argues against oversimplification and dichotomy regarding views of cultural differences between China and Western countries. More specifically, he argues against the popular view that Chinese medical practice traditionally endorses no or indirect disclosure of personal health information to patients, unlike Western medical practice. He argues that China had a tradition of direct disclosure to the patient, unlike some Western traditions, and that the majority of Chinese people today wish to know the truth regarding their medical condition. Nie suggests that this historical and sociological reality is ignored in "the cultural differences argument", which results in the widely accepted stereotype of China as being very different from Western countries in this respect. According to Nie, healthcare professionals in China are in fact making efforts to move toward honest and direct disclosure of the patient's condition. He argues that the shift of attitudes in favour of full disclosure may not be a mere imitation of current Western practice but rather a return to traditional Chinese medical practice. More generally, he rejects cultural stereotypes, and endeavours to explore cross-cultural bioethics with more attention to the normative and shared aspects of ethics and to the complexity and internal heterogeneity of each culture.

In chapter 8, Pyrrho illustrates ethical issues involved in nanotechnology, which may include numerous technological possibilities that may impact on a wide range of industries. What seems troublesome to begin with is the lack of consensus regarding the definition of nanotechnology, other than that it deals with nanoscale particles. More importantly, it concerns the chemical and physical properties originating from the size of these particles. Without more conceptual clarity on nanotechnology, different players understand it differently. Despite inevitable uncertainties, the authors believes that it is important to analyze and discuss potential ethical issues involved in this promising technology before the actual scientific advances take place. They discuss autogenous and heterogenous ethical implications of nanotechnology. The former concerns the scientific consequences of nanotechnology, whereas the latter concerns its bearing on cultural, social, economic, environmental and political matters.

In chapter 9, King, Whitaker and Jones illustrate scientific advances that call for speculations in relation to their potential technological applications. Such technology may involve serious ethical issues. While some speculations may become real in the near future, others may be highly unlikely, such as perfectly tailored prophylactic medication for an individual based on his or her genetic data. Hence, the authors question whether it is worthwhile for bioethicists to engage in speculative bioethics where the issues are based on mere possibilities of consequences resulting from potential technologies. Speculative ethics may be a provocative term. In this chapter, genomic medicine, nanotechnology, regenerative medicine, and cryonics are discussed, with much space given to cryonics as an extreme example involving speculation. Criticism toward ethicists' engagement in speculative ethics relates to epistemological problems and moral consequences of these problems, e.g. being less attentive to current ethical concerns that should be addressed in the present. Still, some critics support the positive role of speculative ethics in guiding the direction of science. The authors oppose such a defense of speculative ethics, arguing that one cannot consider all possibilities and that one cannot determine which possibilities are worth ethical consideration. The authors conclude that bioethicists should be cautious about ethical engagement with speculative matters, although it may not always be easy to discern whether these are scientific facts or fiction.

3. Acknowledgements

Thanks are due to Ian Gallant and Luljeta Pallaveshi for their technical assistance in editing this book.

4. References

Beauchamp TL, Childress JF. (2009). *Principles of Biomedical Ethics*, 6th ed. Oxford: Oxford University Press. ISBN-10: 0195335708, USA.

Rudnick A. (2001). A meta-ethical critique of care ethics. *Theoretical Medicine and Bioethics* Vol. 22, No.6, (September, 2001), pp. 505-517, ISSN 1386-7415, eISSN 1573-0980.

Rudnick A. (2002). The ground of dialogical bioethics. *Health Care Analysis*. Vol.10, No. 4, pp. 391-402, ISSN 1065 3058, eISSN 1573-3394 .

Rudnick A. (2007). Processes and pitfalls of dialogical bioethics. *Health Care Analysis*,Vol.15, No.2, (June, 2007), pp. 123-135, ISSN 1065 3058, eISSN 1573-3394.

2

End of Life Treatment Decision Making

Juan Pablo Beca and Carmen Astete
Centro de Bioética, Facultad de Medicina,
Clínica Alemana-Universidad del Desarrollo,
Santiago
Chile

1. Introduction

Every human being has a personalized life and generates meaning which is subjective and depends on cultural facts, beliefs, faith and biographical experiences. End of life could mean a long period of a human life, but end of life decisions are near death decisions. Death is the loss of biological life and it can be verified. Nevertheless it can be seen as a mystery and is open to different points of views. What is unquestionable is that our human life is finite and therefore it will always come to an end. Death is not only inevitable but a part of each individual life or the last chapter of each personal biography. To be conscious about one's own life's finitude is a unique quality of the human person as a historic and temporal entity. To comprehend its intrinsic dignity and to find deep meaning to human life, it is important to internalize and accept life's finitude and the certainty of death. When this is achieved, it may be easier to die in peace. Callahan says that end of life and death should be more acceptable for those who have accomplished their personal life projects and moral obligations (Callahan, 1995). It is still socially inappropriate to talk about end of life or death. This also holds for physicians and other health care professionals.

Death and dying are not the same. Dying is commonly not a instant but rather variable, complex and frequently lengthy. End of life may take place at any age and may occur because of a variety of physical conditions, chronic or acute illness, degenerative diseases or accidents. Many times dying occurs with much pain and suffering, with a personal emotional and spiritual crisis, anxiety and moral distress. This generates various questions and problems for those who are leaving life and for their loved ones. No matter what their personal beliefs might be, everyone faces the mystery of life and death with doubts or questions that have no definitive answers. This is a perennial issue that is not expected to change with 21st century technology, hence this chapter will not focus on technological aspects of the ethics of end of life.

Most patients at the end of life receive health care, but it is commonly provided without clear objectives and with insufficient knowledge of their wishes and hopes. Care givers are usually very able in their technical skills but confused about what is the best for each particular patient. We are all aware of the many changes in medicine in the 20th century, from earlier when nothing very effective in treating illness could be done, to our days when we are able to cure many diseases and to prolong life for days, months or even many years, although the disease has not been cured. This progress has led medicine to focus on curing and to neglect its historical mission of caring for those who suffer and for those who are in their dying process with the exception of palliative medicine. Many authors have analyzed this divergence of the efforts for curing and for caring. One of the more clear-cut studies was the Hastings Center project to re-establish the goals of medicine (Hanson & Callahan, 1999), where two of the four are: *....cure and care of those with a malady, and the care of those who cannot be cured ... and ......the pursuit of a peaceful death ......* A high proportion of patients at the end of their lives receive treatments that do not benefit them in terms of healing, relief of suffering or personal wishes achievement, and their distress and agony are extended. It is not clear why it has been so hard to improve health care at the end of life.

Situations that patients, families and care givers have to deal with when they care for patients who are at the end of life are numerous and variable. Relevant issues are the need for controlled pain, anxiety and other symptoms; how to know the patient's wishes, fears and hopes; which is the best way to respect his or her values and advance directives if they exist; how to respond to emotional and spiritual needs; how can family and other loved ones be supported; and how can care givers be helped in relation to their own distress. Each one of these and related issues require specific answers and difficult decisions have to be made. There are no easy, precise or general answers. The aim of this chapter is to analyze the complexity of end of life decision making and to suggest some ways to improve it, so that it can benefit patients and their relatives. Four representative situations will be described, to be kept in mind while reading this chapter. Then different types of decisions and related challenges will be discussed, as well as by whom and how they should be made (euthanasia and medically assisted suicide will not be considered in this discussion). Suggestions on how to improve end of life decisions will be made. The underlying assumption here is that the topic is in part an ethical matter as end of life decisions commonly involve conflicts of values, such as prolonging life vs. reducing suffering.

2. Four representative cases

The following situations that are presented raise questions about the end of life decisions that had to be made and the problems that health professionals, patients and family members had to face. Readers should keep these situations in mind while reading through the rest of this chapter.

2.1 Situation 1

A 68-year-old patient who suffered from gastric cancer diagnosed eight months earlier presented multiple peritoneal and hepatic metastases, despite several rounds of chemo and radiotherapy. He was an independent professional, married with two sons, two daughters and eight grand children, all of whom were very close. He understood his disease and accepted his near death based on his strong religious faith. After his last admission to hospital, he decided to be cared for at home and his general condition quickly deteriorated. He was nearly emaciated, despite being on partial parenteral feeding. Four years earlier, due to cardiac arrhythmia that was refractory to medication, the patient had a cardiac pacemaker implanted, regulated to go on if his own frequencies fell below 70 beats per minute. Given the patient's terminal status, some in the caring team expressed their doubts about the pacemaker's effects during his dying process. The patient had mentioned his intention to donate his pacemaker after death, but had not asked for its deactivation. The cardiologists were not sure about the effect of the pacemaker in a possible prolongation of the patient's final time. Nevertheless, they opposed deactivation, which they considered as ethically uncertain. The family was initially in favour of the deactivation, but ultimately decided against it because of the specialists' uncertainty. The condition of the patient progressively deteriorated into a state of stupor and later into a coma. This moribund phase lasted for ten days, with a cardiac frequency invariably fixed at 70 beats a minute, which is explained by the action of the pacemaker. Although physicians and family members decided based on what they felt was the best on clinical and ethical grounds, the patient had an artificially prolonged agony and the family suffered deeply during this period.

2.2 Situation 2

A 46 year old previously healthy industrial manager had a severe car accident while driving alone on a highway. After emergency measures were carried out at least one hour later by the rescue ambulance personnel, he was transferred in extremely poor conditions, unconscious and with visible multiple fractures to a small community hospital. He was intubated and after initial hemodynamic stabilization he was transferred by helicopter to a tertiary care hospital. At admission he was unconscious, with very low blood pressure, severe metabolic acidosis, and rapidly developed multisystemic failure needing mechanical ventilation. His fractures were immobilized and two days later he was connected to dialysis. His neurological assessment demonstrated deep coma, some occasional seizures, and the serial CAT scans showed extensive demyelization lesions and cerebellum and basal ganglia lesions, all of them secondary to a prolonged ischemic encephalopathy. After five days with no change, the neurologists made clear that the patient's recovery would not be possible and that in case of survival he would go into vegetative state or another similar condition.
The patient's wife, his two adolescent sons and his mother were informed about the almost impossible chance of recovery and about the prognosis in case of survival. The possible courses of action, including withdrawal of treatments, were discussed with them and with the neurologist in an ethics consultation meeting. There was neither a living will nor other expressions of the patient's preferences in case of being near death with risk of severe neurological damage. His wife said that she was convinced that if he could choose he would decide to stop all treatments because he would not want to live with such severe neurological damage. The critical care medical staff, although very uncertain about withdrawing treatments, agreed to her demand. After some hours, and giving his family some time to be with him privately and for the administration of sacraments by a catholic priest, mechanical ventilation was discontinued.

2.3 Situation 3

A 60 years old woman was a widow with only one daughter who was married with a two year old son. She had severe disseminated lupus that started many years before, with progressively worsening recurrences. She also had poorly controlled celiac disease and was undernourished. She lived alone and had to sell her small clothing industry as she was not able to run it anymore. Her physical condition had deteriorated because of generalized muscle and joint pain, weakness and extended skin lesions. She became a very isolated person, in spite of having good medical care, well controlled medication, psychological support and the necessary domestic assistance. She had a good but not very close relationship with her daughter, and she had not established a good bond with her grandson. She was admitted to hospital with severe lupus relapse, with pneumonia and in initial renal failure with some signs of encephalopathy. After her dehydration and metabolic state were stabilized and the infection had been controlled she developed progressive renal failure that required dialysis. She was informed that this was a necessary procedure now, which was possibly indefinite in time, and that dialysis could be done as an ambulatory service three times a week. She apparently understood the information but did not agree and refused dialysis. The attending physicians were disappointed, regarded her decision as a result of mental confusion and asked her daughter to decide. The daughter made clear that her mother had for a long time considered her quality of life as very poor and was not willing to accept more treatments, although she had never written a living will nor formally assigned a proxy. She also said that the only other family member that could know the patient's preferences was her brother, but accepted that it was she who had to represent her mother's wishes. She said that she believed that one should fight to be alive but that life cannot be forced by others as an obligation, and that she thought that her mother shared this idea. She consulted with her uncle and the case was submitted to an ethics consultation. Finally she decided to support her mother's refusal of dialysis or any other new treatments, allowing the progression of disease. She said that although it was extremely difficult and sad for her, she had to respect her mother's wishes even if she didn't entirely agree with them.

2.4 Situation 4

This was a 2 ½ year old female infant on mechanical ventilation since her first day of life because of a generalized hypotonia with no muscle reflexes, no swallowing capacity and no spontaneous breathing movements. She could only move her eyelids. She was conscious and could establish eye contact when she was awake. She was fed by a nasogastric tube and several weaning trials had failed.

She was the first baby of a young couple of low socioeconomic and educational level, but they had enough understanding about their daughter's unrecoverable condition. They had established a close attachment and visited her every day in the Children's Hospital ICU.

First muscle biopsies revealed a generalized muscle fiber atrophy which is suggestive of a mitochondrial myopathy. The ethics committee was consulted about treatment limitation and suggested repeating the muscle biopsy in order to have a complete genetic diagnosis as an essential requirement. The committee recommended that only then could a treatment withdrawal be decided with both parents, to allow the baby's death under proper sedation and to provide support for her family. The parents declined consent for further invasive studies or treatments, arguing that they only wanted to avoid all suffering for their baby, that they were not prepared to stop assisted ventilation, and that they ultimately expected a miracle.

3. End of life decisions

Advances in medicine, medical technology, diagnostic procedures, antibiotic therapies, life support treatments and other interventions in critical care medicine in the last few decades have produced many new possible decisions and problems that physicians have to face when they are dealing with terminally ill patients. For each possible intervention or treatment and for each problem patients go through, there are concrete decisions to be made. This is not only a problem in critical care medicine or in the treatment of acute or terminally ill patients, but also when care givers deal with chronic or degenerative diseases at any age, or when elderly people come close to their final stage in life.

In order to consider clinical decisions when a patient appears to be entering the final stages of his or her life, clarity is required in relation to diagnosis and prognosis. After these have been clarified, it becomes necessary to determine if the patient has no real possibility to recover and therefore is in his or her final stage. Only then should end of life decisions be made, focused on what can be regarded as the best for the patient or, in other words, trying to find out what would be the patient's best interest. This is a difficult question to answer as there are many possible ways or courses of action that can be regarded as good and legitimate ways to benefit these patients (recognizing the primacy of patient choice when known).

For each patient who is facing possible death, the amount of care decisions may be numerous, from nursing care and diagnostic procedures to the more complex management or procedures in intensive care. Although a great majority of end of life care decisions involves limiting intensive care or treatments in order to avoid prolonging suffering, we will first note other decisions that should take place before that. The first is the need for clear information provision to the patient or surrogate about his or her condition, diagnosis, prognosis, chances of survival and possible handicaps or extended rehabilitation time needed if he or she survives. This is a problem in itself as it has to be a truth telling process but it also has to be compassionate and appropriate to the patient's emotional and cognitive capacities that are sometimes diminished. In bioethical terms, information provision should balance the patient's right to know and comprehend his or her situation with the physician's duty not to harm him or her by increasing stress or anxiety through inadequate or unnecessary information. Some patients may prefer not to be informed, which should be respected as their right. Occasionally, if the patients are emotionally fragile or partially incapacitated, family members should be asked before informing him or her, at least in some cultures. In other words, this requires kind and proficient communication. Family members or relatives may also have to receive information, but not necessarily the same as the patient. Biographic facts that are private should be confidential but sometimes some family members need to know more details or exact information in order to make their own decisions. Often patients are incompetent because of their prior condition, or as part of the acute state of their disease or treatments, including due to sedation. Sometimes, incapacitated patients will not have appointed somebody as a proxy with a durable power of attorney. Therefore information frequently has to be given to their families as surrogates, as in situation 3, or in relation to pediatric patients, as in situation 4. A complex decision is to establish who can best substitute the patient for his or her decision making. This means establishing who would best know and respect the patient's values and wishes. For this decision it is necessary to be acquainted with the family, with its dynamics and the roles of each of its members, which is commonly unknown when there is no family physician who has known the patient and the family for long.

Before describing specific decisions, it is important to note general decisions that patients and families face. In a terminal or near death situation, should the patient be admitted to a hospital, nursing home, another kind of institution, or stay at home with appropriate care. These are crucial decisions that involve social features, resources and family care and all of them should be based on patient wishes. It is far easier if he or she decides, or when they are incapable if they have formally expressed their wishes through advance directives. In many social groups and cultures, the usual situation is that patients' wishes are unclear or unknown and that their relatives have to express what they think the patients would have chosen. At this stage, physicians are not part of this decision, but they do have the responsibility of treatment planning e.g. if the decision is to care for the patient at home.

The particular decisions to be made at the end of life of patients are mainly related to what is known as "treatment limitations". The first and clearest of these limitations is the patient's refusal of treatment, which is frequent in cases of cancer with metastasis, organ transplant or even kidney failure, when these conditions are experienced as an end of life situation. Patients' rejection of treatment should be considered as right and therefore should be fully respected, based on the principle of Autonomy, unless their capacity is unclear or impaired. The rationale of limiting treatments is to avoid what is known as "treatment obstinacy", which is the approach of doing everything possible to prolong life and avoid death, regardless of its burdens, suffering and costs (Real Academia de Medicina de Cataluña, 2005). Treatment limitation is based on futility and proportionality judgments, which conclude that more interventions will only prolong the dying phase, extending agony and increasing suffering. In different ways, this was the main problem in all four cases presented above. It means not starting any new treatment or procedures, or withdrawing some of them. This cannot be decided in bloc, as each treatment, whether more or less complex, has its own purpose and therefore should also require a particular decision. In these highly sensitive conditions, minor interventions such as an intravenous line, a feeding tube or a biochemical test acquire special meanings for patients and family members. Often, physicians are not aware of these meanings and of the great anxiety that they can produce. It is also important to note that these kinds of decisions are not to be taken as one single and definitive decision, because this is a continuous and evolving process where the patient's condition, symptoms and needs may change every day and even within hours. During the course of this stage, both patients and their families require physicians' and other professionals' support and guidance.

The decisions of treatment limitation usually begin with a Do-Not-Resuscitate order, which means not to do what is routinely established as emergency protocols in cases where the heart stops beating. Another limitation decision, if the patient is already in hospital, is to decide not to admit him or her to intensive care units. Other decisions are to not perform surgical procedures, either major surgeries or minor ones such as gastrostomy or tracheotomy, and not to start vasoactive drugs, antibiotics or other treatments. In these cases, a consistent decision should be to also not perform more laboratory or imaging tests. Other decisions, such as not starting hemo-dialysis or assisted ventilation, are usually more difficult to make, both for professional caregivers and for family members. All these decisions have been described as withholding treatments, but they also can be decisions to stop or to withdraw these or other life support treatments. For many of those involved in end of life decision making, it is more complicated and stressful to decide to withdraw rather than to withhold treatment. Even if the intention of both are in the patient's best interest, and we know that there is no significant moral difference between them, withholding and withdrawing treatment decisions are experienced as different. Perhaps the most difficult (withdrawing treatment) decision is to stop mechanical ventilation, because death may occur shortly after it is performed, and inevitably many will feel it is the cause of death. This was the hard problem faced in situations 2 and 4. Discontinuing assisted ventilation is associated with many fears and myths, such as that it is a sort of euthanasia, or that it is illegal or risky for physicians who could be taken to court for it. In a similar way the deactivation of cardiac pacemakers is a complex and difficult decision as occurred in situation 1. Another special situation that has been widely discussed after the Terri Schiavo and Eluana Englaro cases is the withdrawal of artificial nutrition and hydration (A.S.P.E.N., 2010). These procedures are perceived as a mandatory duty of basic humane care by some or as an unnecessary technical intervention by others.

The decisions described above do not mean abandonment of the patient or that "there is nothing to do". Decisions of treatment limitation can be part of actions that favor the patient's wellbeing, in order to make possible a peaceful death. Therefore, end of life decisions include the planning of efficient symptom and pain control plan with all the necessary medication and sedation.

Other kinds of decisions are related to the patient's spiritual needs, as severe illness and the state of being near death cause a personal spiritual crisis that is frequently unrecognized. Spirituality is understood as the compilation of hopes, fears, faith and values that guide one's plans and meaning of life and death. It involves the spiritual or existential suffering that includes hopelessness, feeling like a burden to others, loss of sense of dignity and loss of will to live. It includes but is not restricted to the patient's religious needs (Chochinov & Cann, 2005; Sulmasy, 2006). The patient's spiritual needs have to be defined by him or herself. But physicians and other health care professionals have the responsibility to make sure that these needs are recognized and evaluated, and that patients are offered the appropriate responses to them. To include spiritual and emotional support as a substantial part of end of life medicine centered on the care of the patient and his or her family will considerably facilitate the patient's peaceful death.

When addressing the topic of end of life decision making, it is necessary to consider that these decisions sometimes have to be made when it is not possible to know the patients' values and wishes. This will always occur in neonates with untreatable conditions, but also in children when their parents have to make decisions on their behalf, as in situation 4. In incapacitated adults because of advanced Alzheimer or other neuropsychiatric diseases, decisions will also have to be made by proxies, but patients' previous values should be respected. Some patients and their families need professional assistance in communication in order that they can better understand their disease and prognosis, and then express their doubts and preferences. This is what is referred to as a guided and assisted interpretive patient physician relation model (Emanuel & Emanuel, 1992).

Decisions for end of life care are influenced by multiple factors related to patients, their families and social environment, cultures, religion, available resources, health policies and more. Decisions may change according to each patient's age, capacity, emotional condition and understanding of diagnosis and prognosis. Decisions may also change if it is a chronic or acute disease and in cases of added complications to previous conditions, even more so if they occur after prolonged admissions to hospitals. Also, decisions are dependent on family fears, hopes, guilt or interests. One should also consider differences between family members' points of views. Decisions related to similar situations may differ in different cultures, for example in Anglo-Saxon, Latin-American, European or Asian environments, where notions about meanings of human life and about death and dying can differ. Cultures influence decisions of patients, families and health professionals. Their religious thinking can determine what they want for themselves or for their loved ones when they are approaching their final stage in life. Whether they believe in eternal life or not, in re-incarnation or in some form of transcendence based on their faith, has crucial influence over their decisions. Decisions also largely depend on the economic situation of patients and families, especially if they have to pay for final care by themselves without state or insurance coverage. Health policies may greatly determine the kind and amount of care people will receive at the end of their life, according to hospital guidelines and available resources. Last, but not least, decisions of quantity and kind of care depend to a great extent on physicians and other professionals' recommendations, which are also influenced by their own cultures, values, experiences and personal sensibilities.

Another crucial issue for end of life decision making is to establish if the care and treatments given to the patient are effective or futile, and if they are proportionate or not. These determinations, sometimes defined as the likelihood of benefit cannot be established as exact determinations. Technical and medical assessment for futility can be based on medical evidence and experience, but proportionality of burdens or costs are non-medical appraisals that should also be considered.

Before describing problems of end of life decisions, it is necessary to define what we understand by euthanasia. Although it is not a focus of this chapter, it is part of an ongoing debate. Different countries and cultures have dissimilar notions, social meanings and legislations about this matter. What many people understand by euthanasia and what some European legislations have approved, refers to well defined procedures to induce death in specific circumstances of terminal patients. The terminology frequently used, of direct or indirect, voluntary or non voluntary, and active or passive euthanasia, causes confusion. Therefore, it is appropriate here to clarify that (medical) euthanasia should only be understood as procedures that intentionally and voluntarily produce the patient's death, because of an incurable disease and unbearable suffering. It is therefore direct and voluntary (Institut Borja de Bioética, 2005). This is different from accepting death as a foreseeable but inevitable consequence of limiting futile or disproportionate treatments in order to avoid suffering and therapeutic obstinacy. The ethical grounding of this is the moral difference between producing and allowing death, and the well known doctrine of double effect. Therefore, treatment limitation should not be confused with euthanasia.

4. End of life decision-making problems

Decisions related to patients who are in terminal conditions because of acute or chronic diseases, as well as to those who are ending their lives with different degenerative conditions, can be difficult and problematic. These problems concern in different degrees patients, their surrogates, physicians and other health professionals. A list of these issues is shown in Table 1. Decisions are focused on patients and their families' views about the meaning of life, the dying process and death itself. In some way, at least in the western world, we live as if we are immortal, not recognizing our finitude. Difficult as it is to admit to any serious disease, it is more difficult if its chances for recovery are rather low. In such a situation many patients go into a personal existential crisis, questioning their life achievements, developing complex fears and hopes. Some of them expect to have time enough to express their wishes, to achieve some reconciliation with family members, to express their gratitude to their loved ones and to pray according to their religion. Other patients, with the same diagnosis and clinical situation, prefer not to know about their condition, and therefore disregard information and deny the illness or its gravity. Some want to extend their lives as much as possible, while others wish to have a short disease, because they accept their death more readily or because they fear the disease and its treatments. A personal approach is required. Imagine a 68 year old male with lung cancer and initial metastasis. His younger daughter is planning her wedding to take place in two months. He will most likely struggle to be alive at least for his daughter's wedding, and then to be able to see her with her new family, hopefully giving birth to her own children. In this situation the patient, his daughter and the whole family will have the same aspirations. In contrast, with the same diagnosis in another patient of the same age, but a widower, retired and living alone, the patient may refuse treatment and expect the course of his disease to be as short and painless as possible. A different situation is that of the parents of a 5 year old son with deep brain damage because of birth asphyxia, who now has a severe pneumonia on mechanical ventilation, with added multiresistant sepsis. Some parents would accept that death, sad as it is, may be best for their child, while others may request disproportionate therapies. Other problematic decisions are organ transplant or abortion decisions, which are influenced or determined by cultures and religions (The Lancet, 2011).

1. Patients' and families' views of death
2. Health professionals' views of death
3. Human life regarded as an absolute value
4. The right to refuse treatment
5. Patients' capacity
6. Surrogate's decision capacities
7. The meaning of the duty to care
8. Quality of life
9. Fears of limiting treatments
10. Specific situations

Table 1. Main issues in end of life decisions

Physicians and other healthcare professionals such as nurses, physiotherapists, and psychologists have views that influence information and guidance for patient or proxy's decisions. Perhaps our own biases are inevitable as we inform patients not only through verbalization but also through our non verbal communication. And these biases in some way determine the emphasis on prognosis, severity of the expected symptoms for the near future, quality of life if the patient survives, and available courses of action (Gilligan and Raffin, 1996). Examples are the issues presented in situations 3 and 4. It is difficult not to be directive when informing patients and their relatives. It is important to recognize that health care professionals are members of the same societies as their patients, although they do not necessarily share the same culture, religion or beliefs. Therefore they may have similar uncertainties and doubts. But it is even more challenging for health professionals, as they may experience the death of their patients as a failure, both personally and of their professions. This is why physicians often feel that even if they cannot cure a patient they have the duty to prolong his or her life as much as possible. As part of the denial of their patient's impending death and because of the difficulties they have addressing family members, intensive care residents try hard to keep patients alive, at least until the next shift. Many times physicians are not prepared to limit treatments, arguing that their role is to prevent death and that they should not play God, by shortening life (although arguably they do so by prolonging life).

Physicians and relatives often excessively prolong the agony of patients. Many end of life treatments unduly prolong suffering. This is therapy obstinacy which is not a benefit but a harm for the patient. A frequent reason to do so is viewing human life as an absolute value. The notion of the absolute does not allow any grades and therefore life should be considered a fundamental and not an absolute value. Still, if or when prolonged agony is worse than death, our moral duty is to avoid suffering rather than to postpone death.

If the above issues are clearly understood, one can recognize and respect patients' right to refuse treatment, which is contrary to the paternalistic tradition of health care. Patients' rights are based on autonomy, which is easier to understand in relation to elective treatments or to informed consent to research. It is more challenging when terminal patients, whose lives can be prolonged, refuse ordinary treatments. This may be because the patient does not want to live anymore in what he or she views as extremely poor conditions, as in situation 3. But it also may be the consequence of fears or of not having full understanding of prognosis and of the treatment, as occurred with the parents' decisions in situation 4. There may be no problem if the refusal is for non-crucial procedures, but serious conflicts might arise when it is for treatments that are considered medically necessary. Imagine patients refusing feeding tubes, drainage or oxygen masks that are simple procedures that mitigate symptoms and do not involve much risk. The conflict may be more challenging if family members agree with these kinds of refusals, but may worsen when family members refuse treatment for patients who have not even been asked about it. In some cultural environments, such as in Latin America, this occurs often because families feel that asking patients about treatment options can be a great emotional burden (to patients) that should be avoided.

Patient decisions about their treatment rely on their right to decide. This right depends on each person's capacity. At times the assessment of capacity will not result in a yes or no answer. If the patient was incapacitated long before the end of life situation, there will be no problem and all his or her decisions have to be made by their proxy. A common situation is that of partially capable patients who now may be less able to understand their diagnosis and prognosis. Other cases may involve previously healthy and normal adults who now have a critical disease with uncertain or very poor chances of full recovery. In these circumstances, although they were previously able to express their desires, they may now not be able to do so. The problem is how to establish whether the patient is permanently or even temporarily incapacitated (Drane, 1985). Capacity implies not only cognitive but also emotional qualities and patients in a critical condition may have some degree of emotional difficulty to make decisions about their end of life treatments (Gilligan & Raffin, 1996). It is necessary to evaluate capacity for each decision in itself. Sometimes patient or family requests appear to be unreasonable or may even be against the law. This would be the case if they demand to abruptly stop all treatments, transfer a patient when it is not possible because of his needed life support requirements, limit treatments when recovery is still likely, ask for the administration of lethal drugs, and other extreme demands. Asking for disproportionate treatments can also be considered as an unreasonable demand. Sometimes asking for more treatment, when there is no chance of recovery and death is likely to occur within the next few hours or days can be considered unreasonable, although it may be understandable. Examples of these situations are demanding ECMO in cases of advanced lung fibrosis, mechanical ventilation in advanced Lou Gehring's disease, or more chemotherapy in final stages of cancer. In all these cases, the conflict between families and physicians may become severe. This should not be seen as disrespect of autonomy but as the limitation of autonomy, because of the patient's partial incapacity or because of unreasonable requirements that would compromise medical integrity.

Assessment of patient's capacity for end of life decision making is not sufficient. Decisions may rely, at least partially, on surrogate decision makers. In some cultures, a proxy can be formally nominated or designated, but in others many family members may honestly think that they have the right to make decisions for capable patients. Stress and anxiety of those who have to decide in the name of their loved ones is strong and unavoidable, which makes it easier for them to avoid treatment limitation choices. Decisions or requirements coming from a spouse, son or daughter who are in severe emotional distress are questionable. Surrogates' cognitive and emotional capacities should be assessed. Decision making may conflict with a family's values, sensibilities and interactions. Examples of these situations are common, especially when one fairly dominant member of a family, sometimes with personal emotional problems or guilt, strongly demands unreasonable treatment or procedures. This can be very common in large families, in cultures where an extended family feels that they can also participate in decision discussions, and in very dysfunctional families. In such cases psychiatric evaluation and support can be helpful.

Other issues concern physicians and other health professionals or caregivers. They all share the moral duty to care. Some of them believe that their responsibility is to always provide all possible treatment to every patient. But the real duty to care is the commitment for the patient's good or best interest, and there are situations where the best for the patient is not to prolong his or her life. Situation 1 and 4 are examples of this. The aim should be not a longer life but a better life. These situations are complex and include many emotions and sometimes severe disagreements among professionals and between them and family members.

The previous paragraph relates to quality of life. Quality of life is a subjective judgment. When somebody says I don't want to live any more, he or she may be saying I don't want to continue living in this condition or with these symptoms. Many people would initially say they would not accept chemotherapy or live with paraplegia or even with a colostomy, but most patients in these conditions want to continue to live. These and other limitations will certainly decrease their quality of life but they cannot be the only reason to withhold or to withdraw treatments. Nevertheless, there are conditions which common and reasonable people would never like to experience. Examples are a permanent vegetative state, advanced Alzheimer disease, severe neurological damage without self consciousness, and patients in unbearable pain with no response to analgesia. Quality of life, even if it is subjective, should be one of the considerations for treatment decisions at the end of life.

Different kinds of patients may require different responses for similar situations. This is so with age differences as decisions on newborns, infants, children or elderly people may differ. Decisions when faced with scarcity of resources, also differ. Imagine deciding to refuse a potentially life saving new surgery, to stop vasoactive drugs or dialysis, to deactivate a cardiac pacemaker (Goldstein et al., 2004 & Mueller et al., 2003) or to withdraw mechanical ventilation (Campbell, 2007). One of the most challenging decisions is the withdrawal of hydration or nutrition in vegetative states. Specific end of life decisions are listed in Table 2.

Treatment limitation decisions
• Do Not Resuscitate Orders
• No more diagnostic procedures
• No more lab tests
• Withholding new treatments
• Withdrawal of hemodialysis
• Discontinuing antibiotics
• Discontinuing vasoactive drugs
• Discontinuing mechanical ventilation
• Withdrawal of artificial nutrition
Patient and family support decisions
• Analgesia and sedation
• Comfort procedures
• Companionship
• Favoring a private room or space
• Emotional support
• Spiritual support
• Family bereavement support

Table 2. End of life treatment limitations and support decisions

5. Who should make end of life decisions?

Up to the second half of the twentieth century, the question who should make end of life decisions had a simple and clear answer. Physicians had to decide, as they were supposed to know what was best for their patient. This paradigm has changed, rejecting paternalism, as patient autonomy has been endorsed. Also, decisions that were few and relatively straightforward are now numerous and increasingly complex because of the rapidly growing number of medical procedures. Nowadays it is not the attending physician who has the power and responsibility for making decisions. Decision making is now sometimes in many hands, each one with their own capacities and limitations (Karnik, 2002). The more agents take part in decision-making, the more chances of conflict which in these highly sensitive situations is difficult and distressing. A list of agents involved in end of life decision making is shown in Table 3.

The default decision maker is the patient, based on his or her right to accept or refuse treatments. This has been socially recognized and established in most contemporary health legislation as part of human rights. The bioethical basis for this is the principle of autonomy, which in health care means that everybody has a presumed right to decide what can be done to him or her, and that nothing should be done to him or her without a formal consent. However, the faculty to act with autonomy depends on capacity, on the full comprehension of the clinical condition, of prognosis and of the possible medical choices. Some patients are not autonomous since they lack minimum capacity, as occurs with infants, younger children, patients who are severely brain damaged, have dementia or are unconscious, and with those who are fully sedated. However, sometimes it may be difficult to determine the patient's capacity. Elderly patients are sometimes treated as incompetent even if they are at least partially capable. Cognitive and emotional capacities are required, as well as freedom, which means the absence of any sort of domination or coercion which also may include some forms of intended compassionate guidance. Patients facing critical disease or terminal diseases are living a personal crisis, and many times feel alone, anxious or frightened. Therefore, their complete freedom to decide autonomously may be questionable. But that doesn't mean that they are not able to make decisions for their treatments and medical care. When they cannot express their preferences competently, other means have to be found in order to fully respect patient values and preferences in end of life care.

- Patients
- Surrogates
- Family members
- Attending and other physicians
- Other healthcare professionals
- Institutional ethics committees
- Ethics consultants
- Institutional authorities
- Judges

Table 3. End of life decision making agents

If the patient is not competent and therefore cannot make his or her own decisions, the best way to proceed is to find out if he or she has previously expressed his or her wish. Although it has been widely promoted in the U.S. and in many other countries, only a minority of people have written living wills where they make known their wishes regarding life prolonging medical treatments, and state the kind of care they would accept or refuse if not able to decide for themselves. These advance directives (living wills) should be known to family members and to caring physicians, but this does not always happen. These documents, although helpful, are not definitive, as they are not very specific and at times only state that the patient would not like to receive extraordinary life support measures or unduly prolonging treatments. Another limitation is that these living wills are established when the patient is not ill and thus is not facing the situation of approaching death. The text may have been written years before and patients could have changed their views or preferences since then. Therefore, living wills should be followed with judgment, as a guide to respect patient values and hence autonomy.

Sometimes patients might have appointed a proxy using a durable power of attorney. Such surrogates have the responsibility to assure that the patient receives end of life care according to his or her preferences. In these cases it is the proxy's responsibility to fully respect the patient's values, and to reject interventions he or she feels the patient would not have authorized if the patient were capable to decide. A surrogate needs to be objective and unbiased, which is not easy as they are usually close friends or relatives who are emotionally involved. The capacity of the surrogate has to be evaluated. When there are discrepancies between medical recommendations and the proxy's choices, problems may emerge which have to be resolved through dialogue.

If the patient is not capable and has not appointed a proxy, then in some jurisdictions it is the family's role to represent him or her in decision making. A difficulty is that many families are large and diverse, so then it becomes necessary to decide who within the family will act as the patient's surrogate. If the patient is married, his or her spouse may substitute unless there is some clear impediment to that. For minor, parents may do so, although there are special problems when parents disagree in their choices or when their wishes are not clearly in the child's best interest (McNab & Beca, 2010). Another problematic situation is that of elderly patients with an absent or incapacitated spouse, and several sons and daughters who may differ in their opinions. In these cases, difficult as it may be to accomplish, it is best to appoint one of them as their spokesperson, making sure that all of them are involved in the decisions that are made. In all these situations, the decisional capacity of those who take part in decision making should be evaluated. Unreasonable requests that are not in the patient's best interest, or that do not respect the patient's preferences, do not have to be followed automatically and sometimes should be discussed and appealed if needed.

The capable patient is the main agent for end of life decisions. A formal proxy or family members are substitutes for incapable patients. This does not mean that patients or proxies are the only decision makers. Historically, physicians were the main decision makers in medical care, which has radically changed in the last decades, but they continue to have an important role in deciding which treatments or procedures will be made available to patients. Physicians have not only the responsibility of providing complete and clear information but also a duty of guidance. Patients or surrogates may not have the capacity to decide by themselves based only on clinical information. They need guidance which means that attending physicians, the different involved specialists and residents, have to suggest the best courses of action. Their guidance has to be non directive and as unbiased as possible; therefore, physicians should acquire and develop these communication and guidance skills (Yeolekar et al., 2008).

There is a wide network of physicians, residents and specialists, which includes intensive care specialists, neurologists, cardiologists, surgeons and infectious disease specialists, among others. This is similar with other healthcare professionals. Nurses are specialized and teams include physiotherapists, psychologists, audiologists, clinical pharmacists, different technicians, social workers and others. Each professional has a distinct appreciation of the patient's problems and what can be done to help him or her in the best way. Not infrequently, patients and relatives establish good communication with the professionals and trust their suggestions. It is common that non medical health professionals and other care providers know more than physicians about the patient's life, hopes, fears and wishes, as well as about relevant issues. These professionals often play a significant role in the decision making process in end of life patients, and this role needs to be acknowledged, encouraged and supported by physicians.

Therefore, the decision making process involves the interaction of several agents rather than a single decision by only one decision maker. This is a crucial notion that will be developed further in this chapter. Depending on the complexities of each situation, more decision agents may contribute to better decisions. When there is a great deal of uncertainty or doubts, and when there are discrepancies between professionals' suggestions and patients' or proxys' wishes, institutional or clinical ethics committees and clinical ethics consultation can be helpful. Ethics committees are multidisciplinary groups whose objectives are to propose guidelines in their institutions, to offer continued education in bioethics for staff, and to analyze complex situations ethically. Situations are presented to committees by physicians, other professionals, patients or families. The analyses are conducted using deliberation, and suggestions are made. The method that each committee uses may be different, but it is important that the method is specified. One of the common methods is principlism, based on how a decision respects and harmonizes the four principles of biomedical ethics: Autonomy, Non Maleficence, Beneficence, and Justice (Beauchamp & Childress, 2001). Another widely used method is casuistic analysis, which emphasizes the weight of clinical facts, quality of life, patient preferences and contextual features (Jonsen et al., 1998). In Spanish and Latin-American committees, a commonly used method is deliberation, as explained by Diego Gracia. It starts with defining an ethical referential frame and continues with the analysis of the clinical situations, the added social or contextual facts, the possible courses of action, and it ends with suggestions and their ethical reasons (Gracia, 2007). No matter which method a committee uses, their analysis should be multidisciplinary, including partners such as diverse health professionals, philosophers, chaplains, social workers, lawyers and more.

Clinical situations with ethical problems occur often in many hospitals, but only a few are presented to an ethics committee. The reasons for this may be that it is time consuming, it may be delayed, and physicians may fear being ethically judged. As a consequence, many informal inquiries are submitted to committee members, who then cannot use a proper method of analysis. As an alternative, individual ethics consultations are used, particularly in the US. Formal ethics consultations are less frequent in Europe and have only been recently reported in Latin-America. Ethics consultations are complementary to the committees and should not replace this institutional ethical deliberation entity. They constitute bed-side clinical bioethics with the purpose of helping to identify and analyze ethical problems of single situations. Ethics consultations, either realized by a single consultant or by two or three members of an ethics committee, assist in decision making in situations with ethical uncertainties, and they can also diminish the moral distress of all involved. Ethics consultation can be conducted by a single consultant or by a team on call. Consultants can analyze each situation with the involved professionals and care givers, with patient families and with patients as much as possible. This has the disadvantage of the absence of multidisciplinary deliberation. Other limitations are that consultations are extremely dependant on each consultant's communication skill, the consultant's biases compassion and tolerance. Therefore, ethics consultants' competencies have been established, in addition to the requirement to be able to comprehend clinical features (Aluisio, 2000). Clinical ethics consultants sometimes become mediators when there are discrepancies between staff, patients', and families' points of view.

Not only patients, surrogates, physicians and other health care providers, institutional ethics committees and ethics consultants have a role in decision making at the end of life. Sometimes hospitals or healthcare institutions have their own guidelines that have to be followed. Health insurance companies may have specific policies that constrain patient care, in relation to assessments, treatment and more. In some countries, some decisions are established by each legislation and in some cases the final decision may be made by judges.

End of life decisions are practical decisions that involve moral judgments. Such applied ethics is uncertain. Some degree of uncertainty is part of many clinical decisions. This may be why clinical and ethical decisions about care are difficult and stressful. So who should make end of life decisions? There should not be a single decision maker. All parties that have been mentioned have a role in the decision making process. Some of them, such as ethics committees or clinical ethics consultants, are expected to use a specific method to analyze situations and to offer suggestions. Decisions are a matter of shared decision making based on an open and tolerant dialogue between all the mentioned parties.

6. How can End of Life decision making be improved?

The question is whether decision making can be improved and if so how. First, decisions should always be focused on what is best for the patient. This means treatment of pain, anxiety and other symptoms, together with fulfilling the patient's needs and wishes as much as possible. End of life decisions should actively pursue a peaceful death. To improve these decisions, it is important to recognize that there cannot be only one method, guideline or decision algorithm, but some suggestions will be offered here.

The focus should always be the patient's "good". This is not a scientific or technical issue. Medical facts are necessary but not sufficient for this. In order to know what is best for each patient, his or her whole biography, values, fears, hopes and preferences have to be considered. Knowledge of social, family, economic and other contextual features is also important. Involvement in decision making of all those who know, love and care about the patient is needed. The aim of end of life care should thus focus on effective palliative care. Decisions should focus on better physical, emotional and spiritual care, and by no means any sort of patient abandonment.

In a strict sense the patient's best interest should be determined by him or herself. This is not possible if the patient is entirely or partially unconscious, which is common when they are in their terminal stage. Therefore the aim is to respect as much as possible what he or she expressed when they were able to do so. When patient have written living wills or have formally appointed a proxy, there is far more knowledge of their preferences, even if the exact conditions or symptoms were not known or anticipated when they expressed their wishes. The basis of this is respect for Autonomy. Hence, a suggestion to improve end of life decisions is to promote that people write their preferences in their own way or using living wills. But, valuable as it may be to have more written living wills, it is even more important that all adults talk about death and dying within their families and, if possible, clarify the care they would like to receive if they have an incurable terminal condition and are not able to decide for themselves.

Another way to improve end of life decision making is to increase ongoing efforts to improve clinicians' communication skills. Their training at undergraduate and postgraduate levels as well as in continuous education programs should develop these competencies that are the basis for getting to know the treatments patients wish for their end of life care. Health care professionals should also be trained to provide emotional support to patients and families. Physicians should also develop their own understanding of the meaning of death, respect the different views that patients and families may have, and acquire the necessary proficiency for symptomatic rather than curative treatment.

It has been suggested that surrogates could be supplied with empirical information on what patients in similar circumstances tend to prefer, allowing them to make empirically grounded predictions about what the patients they are involved with would want (Rid & Wandler, 2010). Relevant anecdotal reports could also be very useful for surrogates. When families take part in decisions on behalf of their loved ones, they will likely have doubts and experience stress. Therefore another suggestion for improvement of the quality of decision making is to support and guide surrogates.

A particularly helpful way of improving family participation in decision making is to provide personal counseling for those who are more involved and to conduct special meetings with the patient's family, other significant others and caregivers. Counseling and family meetings may be conducted by attending physicians or other staff and are typically led by social workers, at least in North America.

Not all end of life situations involve ethics committees or ethics consultants, but the most challenging ones may have a better outcomes if they are consulted. Therefore, a suggestion to improve these decisions in places where there are no clinical ethics committees or consultants is to train in bioethics a group of professionals in order to establish such consultations.

A special and particularly difficult situation occurs when patients who are in nursing homes have a life threatening illness. Whenever possible they should be supported to communicate how they would like to be treated. The majority of people in this situation, particularly in some countries, do not have written advance directives nor have they expressed their treatment preferences. Furthermore, their relatives or proxies may not be available when decisions have to be made. It is not the nursing home staff or caregivers' responsibility to decide what may be adequate and proportionate treatment in each situation. In such situations, it may be helpful to delineate in advance what physicians and non-physician health professionals together with the patient's family regard as the best compassionate care for each patient. If the person is partially capable, his or her capacity should be enhanced if possible, to better know what his or her preferences are. Such pre-determination addresses admission to a hospital or critical care unit, treatment of new diseases or complications, chemotherapy or surgery, artificial nutrition procedures, other support and more. Interesting tools for this purpose are the Physician Orders for Life Sustaining Treatments (POLST) forms that are offered to improve the quality of care that people receive at the end of their lives. POLST are based on effective communication between health professionals, patients in nursing homes and their families. These forms are available in different languages (Oregon POLST program).

Another suggestion to improve end of life decisions is to advocate that they be made in a timely manner, as they are often made after prolonged and avoidable suffering. In order to have these decisions made on time, the possibility of having to make them should be anticipated, preferably at the time of patients' hospital admission or soon after their diagnosis and prognosis have been established.

It is important to remember that end of life decisions are complex and that decision makers will have to take part in lengthy and/or complex processes. It is important to note that everybody involved has specific roles in these processes. Physicians have to determine the diagnosis and the possible courses of action, other health professionals share a role in support and guidance, the patient will have to consent to or refuse treatments, family members or surrogates input the patient's values and preferences (when known), and ethics committees or consultants have expert advising and mediating functions. These are not isolated and independent roles, as it has to be a shared decision making process. End of life decisions will only be (clinically and ethically) good decisions if they are truly shared decisions that respect all points of view in order to fully address patients' best interests (assuming that is primarily determined by patients' capable choices, if known).

7. Conclusion

Advances in medical knowledge, technology, diagnostic procedures and treatment alternatives in the last few decades have produced new clinical and ethics problems, many of them related to end of life decision making. The different decisions to be made at end of life should be based on the patient's best interests, preferences, values and expressions of his or her wishes. With a benefit-burden analysis, the aim ought to be the best treatment for pain, anxiety or other symptoms, and the pursuit of a peaceful death rather than the prolongation of life if that is accompanied by agony (most religions accept reduction of such suffering).

End of life decisions are mainly related but not restricted to withholding or withdrawing specific treatments. The aim is to avoid therapeutic obstinacy and patient abandonment, and to include in end of life care emotional and spiritual support for patients and their families. The process of decision making is associated with different views about the meaning of human life and death, and with patients' and surrogates' rights. Relevant problems are related to the evaluation of decision capacities, differences between caregivers and patients or families, and diverse moral or legal concerns.

Decisions should be made by various agents, including the patient, and proxies or family members as needed. Physicians and the other health care professionals have relevant responsibilities, and ethics committees or ethics consultation have facilitation and mediation roles. The key is that it has to be a shared decision making process with respect for all points of view, addressing what is best for the patient and leaving out other interests (note that justice such as in relation to resource allocation was not discussed here).

In order to improve end of life decisions we suggest: encourage people to write their living wills; support and guide surrogates; and promote timely decision making. In health professional education, clinicians should be trained to acquire adequate communication skills, emotional and moral strength, and at least basic knowledge of bioethics.

9. References

A.S.P.E.N.(2010). Ethics Position Paper. *Nutr. Clin.Pract,* Vol. 25,No.6 (December 2010), pp.672-679, eISSN 1941-2452, ISSN 0884-5336.

Aulisio, M.P.(2000). Health care ethics consultation: nature, goals and competencies. A position paper from the Society for Health and Human Values-Society for Bioethics Consultation Task Force on Standards for Bioethics Consultation. *Ann. Intern. Med.* Vol.133, No.1,(July 2000), pp. 59-69, ISSN 0003-4819 , eISSN 1539-3704.

Beauchamp, T.L, Childress J.F. (2001). *Principles of Biomedical Ethics,* Fifth edition. New York, Oxford University Press, ISBN 0-19-514332-0.

Callahan, D. (1995). *Setting Limits: Medical Goals in an Aging Society*. Washington DC, Gerogetown University Press, ISBN 9780878405725.

Campbell, M.L. (2007). How to Withdraw Mechanical Ventilation. *AACN. Adv. Crit. Care,* Vol.18, No.4,(Oct-Dec 2007), 397-403, ISSN 1559-7768, eISSN 1559-7776.

Chochinov, H.M., Cann B.J. (2005). Interventions to enhance the spiritual aspects of dying. *J. Palliat. Med.,* Vol.8, Suppl.1, S103-15, ISSN 1096-6218. eISSN 1557-7740.

Drane, J. (1985). The many faces of competency. *Hastings. Center. Rep,* Vol. 15, No.2, (April 1985), pp.17-21, ISSN 0093-0334.

The Lancet Editorial. (2011). *Religion, organ transplantation, and definition of death. Lancet,* Vol.377, No.9762, (January 2011), pp.271, ISSN 0140-6736, eISSN 1474-547X.

Emanuel, E.J., Emmanuel L.L.(1992). Four Models of the Physician-Patients Relationship. *JAMA* Vol. 267, No.16 (April 1992), pp. 2221-2216, ISSN 0098-7484, eISSN 1538-3598.

Gilligan, T., Raffin TA. (1996). End-of-life discussions with patients. Timing and truth-telling. *Chest* Vol.109, No.1 (January 1996), pp.11-12, ISSN 0012-3692, eISSN 1931-3543.

Goldstein, N.E., Lampert, R., Bradley, E., Lyn, J., Krumholtz, H.M. (2004). Management of implantable cardioverter defibrillators in end of life care. *Ann. Intern. Med,* Vol.141, No.11, (December 2004), pp.835-838, ISSN 0003-4819, eISSN 1539-3704.

Gracia, D. (2007). *Procedimientos de decisión en ética clínica.* Madrid, Triacastela, ISBN 978-84-9584840.

Hanson, M.J. & Callahan, D.(1999). *The Goals of Medicine. The Forgotten Issues in Health Care Reform.* Washington DC, Georgetown University Press, ISBN 9780878408450.

Institut Borja de Bioètica (Universidad Ramon Llull) 2005. *Hacia una posible despenalización de la eutanasia.*
Available from: http://ibbioetica.org/eutanasia/auta_cast.pdf

Jonsen, A.R., Siegler, M., Windsale, W.J. (1998). *Clinical Ethics,* 4th ed. McGraw-Hill Health Professions Division. ISBN 0-07-033120-0, New York, U.S.A.

Karnik A.M., (2002). End of life Issues and Do-Not-Resuscitate Order: Who Gives the Order and What Influences the Decision. *Chest,* Vol. 121, No.3 (March 2002), pp.683-686, ISSN 0012-3692, eISSN 1931-3543.

Mc Nab, M.E., Beca J.P. (2010). Existen Límites en la Decisión de los Padres sobre el Tratamiento de sus Hijos? *Rev Chil Pediatr* Vol. 81, No.6, pp.536-540. ISSN 0370-4106.

Meisel, A., Synder, L., Quill, T. (2000). Seven legal barriers of end-of-life care: myths, realities and grains of truth. *JAMA* Vol.284, No.19, (November 2000), 2495-2501, ISSN 0098-7484, eISSN 1538-3598.

Mueller, P.S., Hook C.C., Hayed, D.L. (2003). Ethical analysis of withdrawal of pacemaker or implantable cardioverter-defibrilator support at the end of life. *Mayo Clinic Proceeding,* Vol.78, No. 8, (August 2003), pp. 959-963, ISSN 0025-6196, eISSN1942-5546.

Oregon POLST Information. Available from:
www.ohsu.edu/polst/programs/oregon-detalis.htm

Real Academia de Medicina de Cataluña. *Obstinación Terapéutica*. Documento, 2005. Available from:
http://biblio.upmx/download/cebidoc/Dossiers/distanasia0312.asp

Rid, A., Wendler, D. (2010). Can we improve treatment decision making for incapacitated patients? *Hastings Center Report*, Vol. 40, No. 5, (Sept-Oct 2010), pp. 36-45, ISSN 0093-0334.

Sulmasy, D.P. (2006). *The Rebirth of the Clinic. An Introduction to Spirituality in Health Care.* Georgetown University Press, Washington DC, U.S.A. ISBN 15890 10957

Yeolekar, M.E., Mehta, S., Yeolekar, A. (2008). End of life care: Issues and challenges. *J Postgrad Med*, Vol. 54, 173-5. ISSN 0022-3859

3

Ethics Related to Mental Illnesses and Addictions

Barbara J. Russell
Centre for Addiction and Mental Health
and University of Toronto's Joint Centre for Bioethics
Canada

1. Introduction

1.1 Overview

The general public learns about mental illnesses and addictions primarily from mainstream media, including news reports, television programs, and movies. The stories presented usually centre on sensationalism or danger such as those about young women at life-threatening stages of anorexia nervosa or people labelled as "psychopaths." Or the stories appeal to our feelings of sympathy or empathy such as those about people with untreated mental illnesses sleeping on subway vents during winter or a person with moderate dementia who finds greater companionship with someone other than their spouse. These reports and programs often oversimplify the ethical nature of these situations by dramatically pitting one value against another: self-determination versus life, public safety versus rehabilitation, quality of life versus non-abandonment, and happiness versus loyalty. Distilling situations down to one or two values can be motivated more by the ongoing competition for the public's attention and/or economics than by the demands of concise reporting.

However, mental illnesses and addictions are complex, as those who live with a mental health or addiction problem and their families can attest. The high incidence of mental health and addiction problems and their disruptive and lasting impact on people's lives, families' sustainability, communities' well-being, and employers' productivity are publicly acknowledged more often now. In recent years, more and more governments (civic, provincial/state, national) and employers have become interested in listening to those with first-hand experience of these conditions and to those who have developed holistic, integrative ways to diagnose and offer treatments and supports earlier and longer.

Ethical complexity is not limited to crises and strong emotions. It exists in everyday, seemingly routine questions, experiences, and situations. The cases in section 1.2, below, help illustrate the wide diversity of ethically complex, "real world" situations that those living with a mental health or addiction problem, their families and friends, professional healthcare workers and their managers commonly face. Accordingly, the selected cases involve a variety of participants, interests, contexts, histories, health problems, options, and values. The healthcare ethics literature---which is quite extensive now---and educational workshops and courses encourage their readers and participants to increase their understanding of a particular situation or question and they offer various theories, concepts, and approaches to help make ethically defensible decisions. This chapter has similar objectives: first, to broaden and deepen readers' understanding of ethically relevant aspects in living with a mental health or addiction concern; second to increase the understanding of ethically relevant aspects in offering, managing, and accessing healthcare services; and third, to increase readers' abilities to determine which options or responses to a particular issue or situation are and are not ethically sound.

With this said, though, it is not just "soundness" or basic justification that will be emphasized here. Too often decisions can be merely adequate ethically or minimally ethical. The appropriate goal is *strongly* ethical decisions and responses. Whether treating spina bifida, colitis or alcohol dependence, clinicians and healthcare organizations do not talk about providing merely adequate or merely acceptable therapies. In terms of the "technical" aspects of the programs and treatments they offer, their language is peppered with adjectives such as high quality, incomparable, excellent, leading, the best, and world-class. Why then settle for ethically "okay" or ethically adequate analyses and conclusions about these same interventions? A healthcare treatment or service cannot be described as first-rate or promulgated as "the standard of care" if its related ethical features have been simplified or minimized. The level of attention to and engagement with an intervention or service's ethical features directly and proportionately impacts its quality.

Two other considerations contribute to ethically strong health care practices and services. Health and healthcare are not about decisions and choices only. They are also and inescapably about human interactions, whether it is the person's interactions with her family, teachers, or employer, or her interactions with her healthcare team, or the interactions among her interprofessional and interagency workers. In his book, *Ethics and the Clinical Encounter* (2004) and as a philosopher who spends a lot of time in hospitals, Richard Zaner insightfully explores and questions the formal-informal and multivalent-ambiguous interactions that occur routinely between patients and professionals. "How" we are with one another matters a great deal ethically. Arthur Frank, a well-known sociologist whose scholarly interests include the meaning of illness and interactions with professionals and institutions, suggests, "We should speak less of ethics as some activity or substantive content that appears to stand alone and more of *ethical relations*" (2004, 357). In the case of Omar, below, if the defensible option is transferring him to an outpatient program, how this is explained remains important ethically. If the explanation about the pending discharge from hospital and transfer to a community program is condescending, dismissive, and implies the decision is non-negotiable, Omar's defensiveness, anger, and non-cooperation should surprise no one. Unethical language, tone, and demeanour can transform what seems, at the time, to be a good option---all things considered---into a poor and unpersuasive option.

Frank cautions against excessive emphasis on decision making when he states that:

> "Being ethical… has less to do with making a single decision than with initiating a process---often a very slow process---of a person or persons coming to feel that how they acted was as good as it could have been, given the inherent impossibility of the situation (Ibid, 355-6).

Although "inherent impossibility" is meant to refer to healthcare situations typified by complicated machinery, invasive procedures, and life-threatening events (e.g., in intensive care units, in operating rooms, and in emergency departments), Frank's point holds true for long-term mental illnesses and substance use problems, too. Accordingly, this chapter's second noteworthy consideration is participants' characters or who they are, from both the perspectives of important people in their lives and from their own perspective. In modern bioethics discussions and analyses, virtue ethics as an ethical theory has tended to rely on Aristotle's *Nicomachean Ethics* (350 B.C.) and contemporary philosopher Alasdair MacIntyre's *After Virtue* (first published in 1981). More recently, philosopher Lisa Tessman has insightfully examined the durability and praiseworthiness of character virtues in progressively oppressive and harsh situations and societies. *Burdened Virtues: virtue ethics for liberatory struggles* (2005) is a welcome rehabilitation of virtue theory such that it is highly relevant for mental health and addictions settings because unfortunately these settings can be restricting, stigmatizing, and marginalizing.

The remainder of this chapter starts with a description of seven cases and then describes ethically salient concepts and values for mental illnesses and addictions' questions, issues, and situations. Admittedly, some of these concepts are meaningful for any illness, injury or health condition. Nonetheless, certain ethical concepts are especially meaningful for serious mental health and addiction problems. Concluding this chapter by identifying and applying ethical values relevant to each of the opening seven cases might be the expected ending. The experiences of a newly-minted ethicist explain why the actual conclusion is somewhat different.

Daniel Sokol (2007) wrote a perceptive editorial piece in the *BMJ* describing his first days and weeks as an ethicist in a large general hospital in London. Surrounded by innumerable procedures, treatments, and appointments as he accompanies a nephrologist, Sokol observes that, "My proximity to the patients, instead of highlighting the ethical commitments, obscured them" (670). It took awhile before he could see beyond what was urgent and close. With time, he began to see the underlying ethical quandaries, unasked questions, and troubling assumptions. His personal experience underscores an ability or skill that is critical for strong ethical analyses and responses: awareness or discernment (Holland, 1998; Nussbaum, 1985).

In this light, the section on ethical concepts and values is followed by four sections describing other considerations that bear significantly on what constitutes a strong ethically defensible decision or response for mental health and addictions issues and questions. These four sections cover clinical, legal, organizational and systemic factors that cannot be ignored or dismissed by those endeavouring to understand and respond *well* ethically. In healthcare, ethics does not stand alone.... an unfortunate notion that can be reinforced when ethics specialists dramatically "parachute in" to meet briefly with a clinical team and the patient/family and leave just as quickly. Moreover integrating all five aspects means that ethics never trumps everything else (Russell, 2008). It is both naïve and impractical for an ethicist to say, "Just do what is most ethical to do in this situation." Therefore this chapter's concluding section re-visits the opening cases and identifies their ethical, clinical, legal, organizational, and systemic considerations and analyzes what qualifies as strongly ethical decisions and, as per Frank's wisdom, ethically strong interactions and characters.

Stylistic note: Many people consider the term "mental illness" to include addictions. In this chapter, however, they routinely will be referred to separately to ensure that addiction problems are not overlooked. Instead of "substance dependence, misuse, and abuse," the word "addiction" is used to help reduce this chapter's length. Ethical worries about the word will be discussed in section 6.1. Recently, however, various professionals have recommended "addiction" be used in the future *DSM-V*, the diagnostic manual of North American psychiatry. Different words are used to refer to those living with a mental health or addiction problem, such as patient, client, consumer, and survivor. "Client" will be used most often in this chapter because it portrays a reasonable balance in the power and interests between the individual and healthcare professionals and organizations and because most people with these health problems access treatments while living in the community.

1.2 Prototypical cases

The following cases illustrate the ethical complexity of everyday practices and interactions in mental health and addiction settings. It is accidental and unintentional if any case is identical to a real event or person. The cases, however, have been written to be representative amalgams of common situations and issues. All names are hypothetical and used for easier reading and to underscore the human and personal dimensions.

Case 1: Noticing that "Sergei" looks flushed, talks rather loudly and directly, and his breath smells mint-y sweet, the community health clinic nurse asks him whether he has had a few drinks this morning. He chuckles, shifts nervously on the examining table, and says, "Well, not really." "Nothing?" she responds. He looks down at the floor and says "No." This is Sergei's fourth visit for recurring back and leg pain and stiffness. Test results and recommendations from a hospital-based specialist have just arrived. She proceeds to test and document his reflexes, blood pressure, pulmonary-stomach-bowel sounds, heart rate, and temperature.

As she walks down the corridor to see the next patient, the nurse suddenly wonders whether Sergei, who is 46 years old and immigrated with his wife and 2 children from Russia five years ago, drove to the clinic "under the influence" and whether he drinks and drives regularly. She vaguely recalls that he presented the same way at a previous appointment. There is provincial legislation that requires physicians to notify the Transportation Ministry if they believe a patient has a medical condition that makes his or her driving dangerous. The nurse asks herself, "The doctor who will talk with Sergei about the specialist's report… should I tell her about what I am thinking or will she make her own decision when she sees him?"

Case 2: About 2 weeks ago, "Ana Li" was admitted to the mental health unit from the emergency department (ED). Ana Li's mother brought her to the ED because Ana Li was experiencing hallucinations, not thinking clearly, and becoming more and more upset and frenetic. Since admission, Ana Li has resumed taking previously prescribed medications for bipolar disease (she is 19 years old and was assessed as having the capacity to legally consent to treatment). Although she has attended a few of the unit's weekly group activities, sustained or in-depth discussions with her are not yet possible so psychotherapeutic options have not been offered thus far.

During this morning's team review of all their clients, one member mentions Ana Li's continuing hypersexual statements and wishes, and asks whether anyone else worries she will act on them. He suggests her status should be changed from "voluntary" to "involuntary" for awhile and she be restricted to the unit because she may trade sexual "favours" in return for cigarettes from co-clients or someone she meets on or near the hospital grounds. Another team member shakes her head and says, "The Mental Health Act is more interested in preventing major harms like suicide or assault, not casual sex." Another team member immediately adds, "But we have to be realistic about this. Hasn't each one of us remarked how 'drop dead gorgeous' Ana Li is? Plus if there's unprotected sex, then we are going to be dealing with a sexually transmitted disease or even a pregnancy."

Case 3: One of the organization's clinical directors has been working there for almost three months. By introducing new initiatives, he has two goals for today's monthly meeting with the clinical managers and professional heads: (1) to move the program more quickly to the forefront of contemporary mental health and addictions practices, and (2) to be a role model for continuous innovation. One initiative will require at least one home visit for all new referrals in order to understand more quickly and thoroughly clients' individual lived experiences, available supports, and enduring barriers to recovery. The second initiative involves hiring a peer support worker to be a member of each clinical team. Peer support workers serve as unique resources and supports to clients because they have personal knowledge both of living with a mental health or addiction condition and of some of the different ways that family and friends, the healthcare system, the legal system, and social service organizations may and may not contribute to recovery. The director is unsure whether his plans will be met by eagerness, defensiveness, or stony silence.

Case 4: A judge rules that "Jane," who is 68 years old, should not be jailed as punishment for assaulting her landlord when he said she would be evicted in seven days if her apartment remained a fire hazard and malodorous. The landlord fell trying to dodge Jane's fists and a resulting cut required an emergency department visit and six sutures. The judge's ruling diverts Jane to a psychiatric facility for treatment of a mental health condition that results in extreme hoarding behaviour. Review Board hearings are scheduled after the first six months of hospitalization and then every twelve months. Jane is not swayed by her Legal Aid lawyer's advice that she not testify at the first hearing because her nervousness and anger may persuade the Board to not change the order. She testifies and is very nervous, quite disorganized in her responses, and uses some clearly racist language. The Board does not change the mandatory hospitalization order. The next hearing is in one month. Her clinical team believes Jane has improved from her participation in eleven months of behaviour therapy, trauma counselling, and medications, such that they will recommend conditional discharge into the community. Yet a few team members worry that her lawyer will let her testify and her nervousness and inflammatory comments will again persuade the Board to continue the hospitalization order.

Case 5: "Omar" has lived with moderately severe schizophrenia for 30 years; he's now 52 years old. He has lived in different group homes and subsidized housing, has not been close with most of his family since young adulthood, and relies financially on a modest governmental disability program. Omar has inconsistently taken and sometimes discontinued taking various typical and atypical antipsychotic medications for different reasons: the bothersome and discouraging side effects, not wanting to depend on drugs, and simple forgetfulness. Emergency hospitalizations have been required from time to time in order to re-commence or revise medications to reduce distressing thoughts and hallucinations as well as to re-connect him with the community mental health agencies in and near his town. Omar's general health is poor: pulmonary and cardiovascular problems due to chronic smoking and, as a likely result of long-term antipsychotic medications, diabetes, which has been poorly controlled.

Police officers bring him to the psychiatric emergency after finding him asleep in a cold alley on a night when the temperature dips nears freezing. He is hospitalized to resume his psychotropic medications and to try to find a housing facility that offers a modest level of supervision. Since hospitalization, Omar's leg and foot ulcers unfortunately have increased in size and depth despite antibiotic administration. Efforts to keep the ulcers clean and bandages on and clean typically have resulted in arguments between nursing staff and him. The standard of care for the diabetic ulcers now requires debriding and deep cleaning, which will need to done at a nearby tertiary hospital by a specialist. Two weeks ago, Omar agreed to the proposed debridement. On the morning of the appointment, however, he tells the staff member who will accompany him to the hospital, "There is no way I am going to any hospital." Over the next few days, his assigned nurses explain the benefits of the specialist visit and debridement. He eventually agrees again to go because "I don't want to lose my foot." The visit is scheduled for the following week. A week passes. Today when a staff member says "Omar, it's time for us to head over to see the specialist about the sores on your foot and leg," he replies, "No thanks. I don't want someone digging around my foot and leg. I'm staying here."

Case 6: The concurrent disorders (comorbid addiction and mental illness) program is organizing a special day-long workshop to increase community-based physicians', therapists', and addictions workers' knowledge and support for families with a member who has gambling or prescription opioid problems. Four smaller community-based services were invited to help organize the workshop as a way to increase collaboration among the organizations. To attract more physicians, therapists, and addictions workers, two prominent speakers have been invited and the venue will be at one of the area's nicer hotels. Representatives from each partner organization are discussing ways to cover the costs of the hotel's food and beverage services, room rental, and the speakers' travel expenses. Setting the registration fees high enough to cover the costs will likely discourage too many workers at smaller agencies or programs from attending. One of the representatives suggests contacting the regional pharmaceutical representative and a local brewery representative to make a financial donation. Another representative suggests having a raffle for a "fancy spa weekend" as a way to increase the number of registrants.

Case 7: "Sandra" and her partner permit her older brother "Edward" to move into their home while he looks for somewhere affordable to live near his new job. Since she uses many of the household practices they grew up with, Sandra knows her home is a place of comfort and love for him. He promises to see his therapist every three weeks and to have a community physician renew his psychiatric medication before there are only ten pills left. It is important to hear him explicitly commit to seeing the therapist and taking the medications because in the past, he has become so ill that he often verbally abused and threatened those with whom he lived, such as a favourite uncle and his family.

Five months later, Sandra contacts the physician---whose name she finds on the prescription bottle---to ask if crushing the pills into Edward's food decreases their efficacy. She had started doing this two months ago when she learned that Edward had stopped taking the pills because he believed he no longer needed them and subsequently became angry when she reminded him of his earlier promise. Since then, whenever Sandra has found a new prescription slip for the psychiatric medications in Edward's room, she has had it filled by the neighbourhood pharmacist. Yet whenever the physician asks Edward at their appointments whether he is taking the psychiatric medications and feels they are helping, Edwards always says he is taking them as prescribed and they seem to help. The physician refrains from telling him about the conversations with his sister and her actions because he believes that the medications, residing in a home environment, and the sister's involvement are in Edward's best interests.

2. Foundational ethical considerations

A familiar claim by those working as ethics specialists in hospitals and those teaching healthcare ethics is "It's ethics all the way down." Ethics involves what should matter or what should be valued and based on such values, what should be our aspirations, behaviours, and relationships. The word "should" is important here; in philosophical settings, "should" represents the normative element of ethics. There is a critical difference between what is valued and what should be valued. We must ask what are the reasons to value something and whether they are defensible or justified reasons. It is important to underscore that not all values are ethical, though everything that is ethical is based on values. This distinction is often disregarded in healthcare ethics.

Healthcare is informed by a host of values, including self-interest, economics (which can include efficiency and productivity measures), reputation, relationships, and politics (i.e., power). For example, a decision to generate added revenue by charging to train community workers can be justified by economics. To justify it ethically, though, the added revenue would have to be used, for instance, to provide more recreational activities for clients' enjoyment and rehabilitation. If the additional monies were used to increase the agency's profile as the area's "go to" agency, then its justification would be focused on politics and/or reputation. Further examination would be required to determine if a better reputation will or will not contribute to achieving the agency's ethically defensible goals.

2.1 Being humane

It seems obvious that illnesses do not detract from being a human. Yet being a human, that is a member of the *homo sapiens* species, is not the same as being humane. "Being humane" typically means thinking, behaving, and interacting in certain ways. In the context of mental health and addictions programs and services, being humane warrants discussion because it may be what is first sacrificed when units are busy and staff levels are low.

Much has been written in the ethics literature and the nursing literature about the importance of caring and compassion: 21,246 articles and 1,285 articles respectively are listed when these key words are used with CINAHL, a primary nursing database. It is important, however, to distinguish between caring/compassion and respect because they are made manifest by different actions. If a close friend of someone unable to leave his home due to a relapse of his depression arranges an outing that will be as "easy" as possible to accept, this is an act of caring. Prior to deciding whether to go, if the depressed person listens carefully to what has been arranged and why specific arrangements have been made, this is an act of respect. If a case worker has a few toys in his office to occupy clients' children and does not keep clients waiting more than five minutes beyond their appointment time, he has been, respectively, caring and respectful. As Frank incisively points out, "Being ethical… is never anything that one *has*" (2004, 356). It is something one does or strives to do. Skilfulness is relevant to ethics, just as it is to nursing and case management, in terms of astutely discerning what is required and how it can best be accomplished. Ineptness should not be repeatedly forgiven simply because the person had good intentions.

Being humane should also include generosity and welcome, two qualities often overlooked in everyday interactions. Generosity is not about money. Instead it is a philanthropy of spirit and hope wherein people are pro-the Other. Yet this generosity does not equate to strident self-sacrifice and Puritanism. It involves giving but it can be in small, subtle ways. While generosity is a giving or contributing to, without expectation of return, welcome is a taking in wherein the presence of the Other is appreciated. The history of mental health and addictions work and settings includes far too little generosity and welcome. This constitutes an ongoing challenge for contexts in which police powers can be employed: how to once again be seen as generous and welcoming after a client has lost some basic civic rights and freedoms (e.g., involuntary hospitalization, use of a seclusion room)? Welcome and generosity can fade in the wake of efficiency measures, bed flow pressures, staff shortages, and management by statistics; operations may improve economically, but not ethically.

Finally, being humane means relationships are inescapably important, given that human beings are social creatures. In health care settings, ongoing attention must be paid to honouring and maintaining appropriate boundaries between clients and staff. This can be especially challenging because workers utilize various methods to examine and influence highly personal and intimate aspects of clients' behaviours. Moreover clients may not have many affirming and reliable relationships, often due to their illnesses' symptoms, which, in turn, cause family and friends to disengage. Healthcare workers may believe compassion justifies them filling this relational void by taking on the role of friend, family, or confidante. This erroneous belief increases the likelihood of enduring boundary crossings or repeated boundary violations. It is not surprising that medical and nursing books and curricula routinely discuss maintaining appropriate professional relationships and avoiding inappropriate personal relationships, boundary crossings and boundary violations.

Being humane can be most challenging when staff work with individuals who are diagnosed as having a personality disorder. While the resulting behaviours seriously test the therapeutic alliance, too often the label of "difficult client" or "difficult patient" predetermines all activities and it becomes a self-fulfilling prophesy (Hilfiker, 1992; Knesper, 2007; Lauro et al., 2003). In the case of those diagnosed with sociopathy, public rhetoric has often labelled these people as "criminally insane." Since they appear not to be motivated by common morality, these individuals may be judged to be less than human. When working with clients with personality disorders, healthcare workers must avoid such moral judgments. Healthcare and health professions' mandate is to help preserve and restore health and well-being and alleviate suffering, irrespective of inferences about a person's goodness or badness (Pouncey & Lukens, 2010). With this said, though, employers must provide effective forums and measures to alleviate a worker's fear of a specific client and to prevent or address dislike of or negative feelings towards certain clients (e.g., someone convicted on infanticide). The concept of countertransference is well-known in the psychiatric and psychological fields. It is a professional's response to a client's behaviours or statements such that the professional shifts into an inappropriate role (e.g., parent, disciplinarian, rescuer). Psychiatry and psychology textbooks and courses teach ways to prepare for, recognize and effectively address countertransference. Similar attention to the psychological responses of other allied health workers is needed because their negative (or sometimes unchecked positive) feelings and attitudes can obstruct clients' recovery.

2.2 Being a person

Personhood or being a person is a longstanding concept in academic communities, regardless of whether it is political science, sociology, theology or moral theory. Much debate has been generated because of its political, legal and ethical significance: those who legitimately qualify as "persons" must be accorded a certain level of attention, respect, and assistance while "non-persons" can be accorded less. Various philosophers have developed different definitions of personhood. For instance, British philosopher John Locke held that a person was a being with a complex, psychological conscious that continued over time. Focusing on consciousness, cognition, and affect meant that as time passed, people with progressive dementia would become different people compared to their former selves and when certain defining abilities faded, non-persons. Alternative definitions have been offered; for example Rosfort and Stanghellini hold that personhood is "the identity of an embodied self, which is embedded in a coexistence with other selves through time" (2009, 286). Grant Gillett (2002) appeals to a cumulative and evolving narrative of "my life" while Bruce Jennings (2009) posits the "memorial person" wherein someone with advanced dementia remains a person and connected with her earlier years through the memories of those around her.

Farah and Heberlin (2007) present various theorists' definitions of personhood to demonstrate that consensus in defining such a potent concept still does not exist yet. In fact, Tom Beauchamp (1999) recommends discontinuing efforts to refine the moral or metaphysical attributes of personhood. He favours working on concepts that more directly capture the lived reality of daily life. In the case of mental illnesses, clinician, family, employers, and the general public's interest can be focused on psychiatric diagnoses, impairing symptoms and behaviours so much that individuals are de-personalized. Hospital and governmental agencies' operational and administrative practices can depersonalize, too.

De-personalization is ethically indefensible because the individual is not recognized as unique (Peterneliji-Taylor, 2004; Sierra et al., 2006). Instead forms and computer programs can average or homogenize clients such that they become "another case of X" or as Flanagan et al. note, "the medical chart." De-personalization silences such that the individual's unique perspective, lived history, and hard-won expertise are not sought or are ignored. Moreover "othering occurs in relationships between the powerful and the powerless, where vulnerabilities are exploited and where domination and subordination prevail" (Peterneliji-Taylor, 133). French philosopher Emmanuel Levinas' work counters de-personalization by morally and positively privileging the Other and his presence-to-me (Burns, 2008; Nortvedt, 2003; Standish, 2001). Simply put, if I am in the presence of someone else, I am automatically and inarguably obliged to respond to him and respond in certain ways.

Respect is one of the most popular concepts employed to avoid de-personalization in mental health and addictions settings. Too often, however, determining what actually demonstrates respect in a particular situation with a particular person or group of people receives scant attention. Instead a kind of basic civility is considered sufficient. But it is not, especially when healthcare institutions and clinicians are expected to provide high quality treatment and care. Preventing de-personalization of individuals with mental health and addictions problems requires Levinas-ian active engagement with them and equal acceptance plus a kind of existential attention and presence. Processes for information disclosure, clinicians' truth telling, and obtaining informed consent can dominate routine interactions with clients and their families such that little consideration is given to clinicians and staff *being with* clients and families. The effect is eroded personalization of clinicians and staff as well as of clients and families. In other words, healthcare workers also become interchangeable, "all the same," and regrettably for those they serve, forgettable.

2.3 Being a member of a community

In mental health and addictions, considerable focus is paid to people's rights and freedoms. This makes sense because it is so common for others to intervene to limit individual freedoms and obstruct the exercise of rights. Ethics related justification for such interference typically comes from safety concerns, either for the individual herself or for others. However a hidden, but common, concern is the existence of double standards wherein those with suspected or diagnosed mental health problems are not permitted to do certain things while the rest of society are. Some examples help make this point. Restrictions on sexual and intimate activities between hospitalized clients are often excessive. The only permitted activities are those deemed socially responsible, such as not engaging in "casual sex" or "risking a pregnancy." And yet a common freedom is for people to decide how sexually active they will and will not be. Moreover women are permitted in many countries to seek an abortion, especially before the third trimester, so it is discriminatory to summarily hold that women with mental health concerns must always act so that pregnancy avoided. A more ordinary example of double standards involves medication regimens. Exercising, eating balanced meals, getting sufficient sleep, and drinking enough water contribute to feeling and performing well. Most people do not engage in such activities consistently. In general, people are non-compliant. Yet those who have mental health problems are expected to be highly compliant with their medications and non-compliance is summarily often assumed to reflect abnormally impaired thinking abilities and motivations.

The notion of citizenship moves people with mental illnesses "beyond the mere allocation or management of financial or physical resources and implies instead a form of moral assistance that calls for their full participation" (Perron et al. 2010; 108). Rights and freedoms associated with citizenship are ethically very important. But what is often disregarded is whether a person belongs within general society and within different sub-groups that are meaningful to him. Belonging here emphasizes that the person is a valued and equal member such that if he is absent, he is missed and he owes other members certain things just as they owe him. He is accepted "as is," both in terms of recognizing inescapable human fallibility, inconsistency, strengths, aspirations, and all that has led him to be who he is here and now. This goes beyond emphasizing the provision of quality services to those with mental health and addiction worries. Citizenship and belonging focus on membership within a particular network of relationships. Discrimination and marginalization can result in the person being "not of us" and outside the community or relegated to its impoverished and lonely margins, both of which are existentially cruel.

Another often overlooked communal factor focuses on expectations. Too often the general public expects too much of people with mental illnesses and addictions because they do not give adequate weight to the impact of the social determinants of health, stigma and the often discouraging chronicity and relapse of these illnesses. On the other hand, society can be overly paternalism and sympathetic such that too little is expected. Opportunities are not taken to encourage and applaud people's perseverance, kindnesses, resourcefulness, and lived expertise. Instead focus can be merely about psychological and behavioural symptoms of the illness and the prescribed therapies and treatments, not about the kind of person he is.

He becomes defined by the illness. This ethically troubling reductionism explains why many eschew language such as "he is autistic..." or "schizophrenics are..." and instead speak about "those who are living with depression" or "he has a borderline personality disorder diagnosis or traits."

2.4 Being a caregiver/provider

There is empirical evidence that family and friends provide significant assistance and support for those with mental health and addiction problems. This often presents practical challenges if applicable legislation regarding personal health information prohibits disclosure to family members without the client's explicit consent. In most instances, mental illnesses are not yet curable; they are long-term health concerns. This means that family and friends are even more important in supporting someone through expected relapses. Some of these relapses can be highly damaging to these relationships: for instance, dementia often results in aggressive behaviours as well as dis-inhibition (e.g., undressing, frequent swearing, sexual remarks). Mental illnesses can result in frightening behaviours such as verbal, psychological, and physical aggression, loss of property (e.g., if a person has gambling problems or drives while impaired), and more. Therefore, family members may require emotional and psychological help to deal with their fears and distress as to the shared impact of the person's mental illness or addiction. Family members can become secondary "sufferers" of a particular illness or addiction.

The unique nature of psychiatrists' and therapists' work "[places] additional ethical demands on practice" (Radden & Sadler, 2010, 59). Meaningful therapeutic engagement requires entering into the inner lives of clients, examining and often times challenging clients' interpretations, beliefs, self-image, fears and hopes. Clinicians may learn details that no other person in a client's life knows. In the name of safety, healthcare workers are permitted, often expected, to use governmental or police powers that will violate fundamental rights and freedoms. Accordingly, professionals' characters are very important. Radden and Sadler identify a considerable number of characterological virtues and offer detailed explanations as to why they are essential to the routine or everyday work of psychiatrists and therapists. The needed traits include trustworthiness, self-knowledge, integrity, empathy, warmth, sincerity, authenticity, unself-ing, "respect for the patient and the healing project," and more (Ibid, 136).

In forensic settings, a common concern is divided loyalties wherein professionals and healthcare teams are expected to prevent the individual from harming others and violating civil or criminal laws, and yet work with the person to build a therapeutic alliance to help recover from the illness or disorder. When clinicians are asked to assess a person for the court's purpose, it is essential that the person understand that the clinician is acting for the benefit of the court, not for her benefit. In this case, the overarching fiduciary responsibilities of physician-client or nurse-client are suspended to a certain extent. If the psychiatrist or therapist is unable to have a different relationship with the client in doing this assessment, it is ethically wise for him to decline to do the assessment. The general public often does not appreciate the inherent tensions between healthcare systems' and clinicians' roles and the judicial system and lawyers'/police roles, especially when the public's fears and biases are exploited by the media or by political interests. Yet the value conflict between these two systems is ethically necessary, as discussed in the sections below.

3. Why science, technology, and clinical factors matter ethically?

Compared to many physical medicine interventions and programs, mental health and addiction services and treatments face added challenges that have ethical import. The following three issues clarify these challenges.

3.1 Our knowledge about mental illnesses and addictions

As Schmidt et al. note, "Definitions of mental illness tend to contain two aspects: a normative element and a functional element. Normative definitions delimit abnormal behaviour in light of what is typical, usual, or the norm.... [while] maladaptation suggests some diminished capacity to function relative to the average" (2004; 10). Yet authoritative statements of knowledge and fact are fewer in psychiatry and psychology than in physical medicine. Individual experience and subjectivity still inform most psychiatric diagnoses. Scientific uncertainty continues, as illustrated by briefly describing the evolution of psychiatric classifications.

In 1948, the World Health Organization created the *International Classification of Diseases* (*ICD*). In 1952, the American Psychiatric Association (APA) published the *Diagnostic and Statistical Manual of Mental Disorders* (*DSM)*, a short glossary of different psychiatric disorders based on psychoanalytic theory. This was considered a positive first step because various disorders were identified and publicized for the practice community's use. Yet the *DSM-I* was not widely embraced because the disorders were relatively broad, the descriptions quite brief, and many practitioners were not Freudians. Sixteen years later, *DSM-II* was published, but the changes did not significantly resolve the first version's limitations. However *DSM-III* (1982) was different. It was reputedly not theoretically grounded. Instead, its diagnostic categories were based on observed and reported behavioural symptoms. It garnered praise from the psychiatric community because its multiple axes of contributing problems represented the disorders' complexity more accurately. Moreover, the categories and diagnostic criteria had higher inter-rater reliability (Pincus & McQueen, 2002; Schmidt et al., 2004; Wilson & Skodol, 1994). *DSM-III-R* (1987) included various clarifications and corrections. While *DSM-IV* (1994) was much like its predecessor, how it was created was particularly noteworthy: expert teams' consensus about each disorder was augmented by input from the psychiatric community at large as well as those involved in revising the *ICD*. *DSM-IV* also was based on scientifically stronger empirical (as opposed to anecdotal) evidence. Although *DSM-IV-TR* (2000) reflected no major revisions, it did provide various clarifications.

During this period, an anti-psychiatric movement emerged in the United States. One of its best known proponents is the psychiatrist Thomas Szasz (2009; 1976; 1961). He contends that very few disorders are brain-based or organic. Instead, the majority of *DSM-IV* disorders reflect personal preferences that do not comply with social norms. As a result, these people experience difficulties in daily life. Those who feel that the harms of "mis-fitting societal norms" outweigh the benefits can, if they wish, seek assistance from other people to reduce or eliminate such difficulties. But since the maladies are not physiological, says Szasz, it makes no sense to seek physicians' and medical programs' assistance.

The anti-psychiatry movement endures today. In fact, some individuals and advocacy groups embrace the term "madness" as one way to counter what they believe is psychiatry's and medical institutions' illegitimate and hegemonic power and authority (Foucault, 1988; Wilson & Beresford, 2002).

The epistemic process of typological knowledge creation is often called nosology, or medical classification/categorization. Nosology continues to be an issue in mental health and addictions work because the questions still remain: "What makes something a mental [or addictive] disorder? and, Does this something form a category?" (Schmidt et al.; 11). In 2012 or 2013, the APA will publish the *DSM-V*. It will include a new framework or approach: dimensions, rather than mainly categories. There will be two general kinds of dimensions. First, clinicians' diagnoses will take into account the severity of symptoms, rather than mainly their presence or absence. Second, there will be "cross-cutting" symptoms, such as anxiety and suicidality, which occur in many illnesses. As a result, some disorders are expected to be de-listed and some new ones listed. In other words, some people will no longer have a psychiatric diagnosis, some people's diagnoses will be refined, and some will be newly diagnosable. Professional debate about the advantages and disadvantages of this new approach has been pronounced (Banzato, 2004; Collier, 2010; Helzer et al., 2007; Kraemer, 2007).

A similar debate is in progress in addiction treatment and care. Is an addiction to alcohol, tobacco, illegal drugs, or prescription drugs some type of disease, or a personal choice, or something else? The most popular alternative to the disease paradigm considers addictions to be more complex: they are the combined result of biological, psychological, and sociological factors. Researchers and practitioners differ as to which paradigm they believe is most accurate. But the ethical implications of this difference are real. People who develop cancer, psoriasis, or glaucoma are generally not considered ethically culpable for the loss of important abilities or for requiring publicly funded health services. If alcoholism is deemed to be a disease, then the alcohol dependent person may not be blamed for "having it." This is a welcome correction to the traditional moral condemnation of people with drinking problems. If responsibility follows causation, then a biopsychosocial explanation presumes something different. People's physiology, psychology, and social environment are presumed to be self-controllable and modifiable, albeit not totally. They are also presumed to be modified by other people's actions and inactions. Accordingly, if there are negative consequences, culpability for what could have been changed must be shared, rather than resting solely with the individual. The locus of responsibility relative to having an addiction matters ethically because it connects with the ethical concept of fairness. This concept of fairness, and more specifically equality and equity, helps determine the amount of publicly funded versus privately funded services individuals with an addiction problem should be able to access.

3.2 Treatment and care

Those who are not psychiatrists, psychologists, or addictions therapists may not realize how very diverse available treatments and therapies are. For instance, there are more than two hundred psychotherapies, clustered, for example, as cognitive behaviour therapy, family therapy, mindfulness, art therapy, psychoanalysis and more. This increases the uncertainty and complexity of finding the therapy that will benefit a particular person most or at least sufficiently. In the case of psychopharmacological treatments, they have had a checkered history. In the 1950s, new medications were hoped to provide effective and sustainable relief of illnesses' disabling symptoms... a promising change from the seeming unending-ness of psychotherapeutic counselling and from the irreversibility and extreme invasiveness of psychosurgeries. In addition to the physiochemical benefits, medications could also be administered without a client's cooperation or consent. This was not possible for psychotherapies. They could not be beneficial if the person was not in the appropriate stage of change and was not willingly engaged, irrespective of whether she or a substitute decision maker had consented.

The first generation of antipsychotic medications or "typicals" unfortunately caused too many people very serious and irreversible side effects such as tardive dyskinesia. The next generation of antipsychotic medications, the "atypicals," were expected to cause fewer side effects. While second generation drugs have helped many people, the long-term effects are discouragingly negative. For instance, individuals diagnosed with schizophrenia may develop diabetes due to some of these medications (Amiel et al., 2008; Lowe & Lubos, 2008; Muench & Hamer, 2010). Yet it takes years and millions of dollars to develop a new pharmacological treatment that can offer meaningful improvements, not just in terms of biochemical or physiological measures, but in terms of quality of life measures as well. The negative effects of medications, such as significant weight gain, slowed thinking, and sluggishness, help explain in part why people discontinue using them, only to find that they relapse into a serious state that may require emergency or involuntary hospitalization.

From the outset, funding of research of mental illnesses and addictions has been disproportionately low compared to funding of research of physical illnesses. In 2004-2005, for example, the Canadian Institute of Health Research devoted 7.5% of its $700 million budget to mental health and addiction (Senate Standing Committee, 2008). Yet approximately 20% of Canadians have a mental health problem during their lives. In the same year, the U.K. spent 6% of its £ 950 million governmental health research funds on mental health (Kingdon & Nicholl, 2006). In 2011, the American National Institutes of Health will allocate only 4% of its budget to the National Institute of Mental Health (National Institutes of Health, 2010). Consequently, available treatments and therapies are often less reliable and less specific than those for various medical problems. Moreover, more research funds are spent on pharmacological interventions compared to psychotherapeutic or alternative interventions, in part because the pharmaceutical industry spends almost as much as governments on healthcare research (World Health Organization, 2004). This means that new or more effective psychotherapies are less likely to be developed and that a proportion of research funds are used for economic purposes, namely improving a medication's competitive marketability and profitability.

3.3 Daily practice models

Different clinics and hospitals offer markedly different addiction and mental health treatments and programs (Finney & Moos, 2006; Futterman et al., 2004). For instance, one addictions program's work may be guided by harm reduction principles. Familiar examples of a harm reduction approach are safe injection sites and methadone maintenance programs for ex-heroin users. Another program's work, however, may be guided by an abstinence model of treatment. Furthermore, what counts as harm reduction can differ considerably among clinicians (Miller et al., 2008). They may calculate the benefits and harms of a particular activity differently; for instance, providing information about different settings for alcohol consumption and their relative risks. Just as importantly, though, clinicians' opinions may differ regarding the morality of said activity. For example, accepting a client's decision to begin taking taxis during weekend drinking binges as harm reduction may seem to condone the client's wilful drunkenness. Some clinicians believe this clearly violates their professional ethos; others do not (Miller; 2008).

Models of care for mental health settings are also diverse: for instance, strengths-based, empowerment-focused, recovery, trauma-informed, custodial, rehabilitative, and sanctuary. As a result, how clients are seen and engaged by clinicians and teams will vary. A strengths-based approach, not surprisingly, attends to clients' positive abilities to deal with and improve their health and circumstances. An empowerment approach emphasizes correcting historic and current power imbalances---typically profound imbalances---between people with a mental health or addiction problem and professional caregivers and their institutions or between these same people and society at large. The ethical concepts of agency, self-determination, voice, and liberation resonate with empowerment. A recovery approach focuses on a person's valuations, aspirations, interpretations, and pace and it adopts "the long-view" wherein recovery is acknowledged to be an ongoing and unfolding journey. As shown in Gagne et al. (2007) and Ontken et al. (2007) in relation to recovery, focal ethical values are narrative integrity, resilience, commitment, and fallibility.

It is ethically important to identify and understand the practice model relevant to a particular treatment situation because inherent ethical values can vary. In terms of a specific program's model of care, an ethics-related goal should be coherence among the model's foundational values, staff-client interactions, and the kinds of therapies and care offered. However, models can become out-dated as more is learned about what helps clients maintain and regain important activities and relationships, as other programs and systems change, and as certainty increases regarding what qualifies as mental illnesses and effective interventions.

Psychiatry, psychology, and case management qualify as "forensic" when they are applied to and used in our justice system. These include scientific and theoretical analyses of criminal behaviour, clinical and institutional/communal efforts to prevent or deter law-violating behaviour, risk assessments and diagnoses for judicial proceedings, and police psychology. Ethically critical to this work is separating understanding why a person behaved in a certain way---in terms of "nature and nurture"---and morally judging him or her. Conflating nature and nurture or conflating biological processes and socializing processes typify anti-psychiatry's worries.

4. Why law and regulations matter ethically

It is sometimes said that mental health and addictions services and settings are dictated by laws and legal institutions, be they the courts, legislatures, regulatory agencies, prisons and jails, or the police. A common concern is that society uses its various powers for its collective interests to the detriment of individual or minority interests. This concern is historically accurate in many countries in terms of how they have responded to individuals with mental health or addiction problems. Too often, these responses were dictated by social norms for acceptable behaviours and appearances. If the behaviours or appearances violated these norms and rules, common responses were punishment, social expulsion, controlled quarantine, surgical interventions, and even death. However, there were often compassionate individuals and religious-based groups that countered societal edicts by offering agapic assistance and places of sanctuary to people seen as innocent sufferers of cravings or disordered thinking.

4.1 Rights and duties regarding decision making and consent

Personal decision-making typically is one of the first ethical concerns in healthcare settings or issues, in large part due to the courts and legislatures. Today, healthcare involves many therapies and procedures, even in economically disadvantaged or developing nations. Most medical and nursing training programs now include seminars and discussions about clients' legally-protected rights to start, modify, or discontinue any intervention or service and the ensuing duties of professionals to honour such decisions. Valid consent---which authorizes a professional to act---is obtained when the person is informed about the particular intervention's benefits, risks, and burdens compared to other options, has the requisite capacity to make this decision, and is not being pressured, coerced or manipulated to decide.

These three components of the consent process can be obstructed or compromised by the nature or symptoms of mental illnesses and addictions. First, being informed. Healthcare workers frequently overlook this component when clients decline recommended treatments. This is why the consent process is shared: if a treatment is declined, the reason may be that personally irrelevant, non-meaningful, or unintelligible information has been unintentionally provided. Timely disclosure and intelligible explanations are among clinicians' routine duties. As per the clinical section above, our understanding of the nature and causes of mental health and addiction problems is relatively limited, though it is increasing. Accurate diagnoses can take considerable time and prognoses may be quite uncertain. Available therapies and treatments may be scientifically promising, but still lack sufficient high quality research studies to be able to provide highly reliable and nuanced details to patients. Consequently, clinicians can find it difficult to provide clients with individualized and useful information about their illness, prognoses, and personally beneficial treatments.

The second component of a valid consent process is having "enough" mental capacity to decide. When clients decline treatments, this component can garner disproportionately more attention from clinicians than the other two components. Governmental legislation often stipulates specific criteria that, if not met, mean the person lacks the legally required abilities to make his or her own health-related decisions. Two criteria often comprise legislated standards: (1) is the person able to understand the information, and (2) is he able to appreciate the consequences of having versus not having the intervention. These abilities can be undermined by mental illness or addiction. But no set of assessment questions or exercises qualifies yet as *the* validated set for accurate assessments. Consequently, different clinicians may assess a person differently in terms of having or not having capacity for a particular decision. Importantly, however, legislation and court rulings typically hold that someone who has a mental health or addiction problem can *still* have the needed capacity to consent to or decline a recommended therapy. In other words, depression, mania, paranoia, or hallucinations do not, in and of themselves, void the needed abilities to make treatment or other health-related decisions.

The third component is voluntary-ness. Certain therapies and care can involve social, environmental, and bodily control (e.g., group counselling, behaviour modification, protective devices). Coercion therefore is an ongoing possibility. Moreover, some mental health problems can result in a lack of self-control (i.e., mania, dis-inhibition) or in heightened fears (e.g., paranoid schizophrenia, having a history of trauma or abuse). This means that the invasiveness, demanding-ness or restrictive-ness of certain treatments may be very unwelcome, even though they can benefit the person in other ways. Furthermore, despite an appropriate substitute decision maker consenting to treatment on behalf of someone lacking capacity, it will still be traumatic and damaging to the therapeutic alliance whenever a treatment is administered against the person's will (e.g., with Security staff present, by forced injection, by forced application of a protective device to prevent self-injury). Accordingly, before deciding whether an intervention fits with the person's prior expressed wishes and best interests, a substitute decision maker must understand not just the type of treatment recommended, but also how it will be administered and what will be the individual's likely experience of "being treated."

4.2 Rights and duties regarding privacy and confidentiality

Governmental legislation about the collection, use, and sharing of personally identifiable health-related information is common today. These acts, statutes and regulations protect citizens' right to privacy regarding their health, minds, bodies, and related activities by delineating professionals' and organizations' duties to keep such information as confidential as possible and yet use it effectively and efficiently. To preserve clients' and families' trust, limits to confidentiality and any legally required duties to report should be discussed as early as possible by healthcare workers. Later in this chapter, stigma and discrimination will be discussed in detail but suffice it to say that the need to protect mental health and addictions related information is especially important. The consequences of a person's employer and insurer learning that he or she has or has had a mental health or addiction problem can be significant and irreversible. This need to protect this information, however, can unintentionally frustrate, even damage, professionals' interactions and relationships with patients' families.

While many healthcare organizations include family-centeredness among their corporate values, this is more complex in mental health and addictions settings because family may have knowingly or more often, unknowingly, contributed to the person's poor health. Too often, family members emotionally, psychologically, and/or physically abuse one another. Yet research and testimonials show that people recover and sustain a good quality of life because of familial support. More strongly put, family support can be a protective factor (Cleveland et al. 2010; Ivanova & Israel, 2006; Korol 2008; Piko & Kovacs, 2010). Negotiating this quandary requires healthcare workers to have strong communication, interactive and assessment skills. Clinicians and healthcare organizations must be proactive in instituting practices to safeguard clients' privacy and to balance the competing interests of clients and their families without losing their trust or compromising their relationships further.

4.3 Rights and duties regarding safety

The political philosophy concept of *parens patriae* means that a legitimate government serves much like a patriarchal parent or father to its citizens. It is thus responsible for their general well-being and safety, and at times must make decisions that contravene their immediate wishes. A citizen may be in danger of being harmed such that those formally delegated powers to fulfill the government's duty (i.e., such as police and medical professionals) are expected to intervene on his behalf. So too if the citizen is harming or posing a serious threat to another innocent citizen. Governmental representatives may act unilaterally to stop or prevent such harm, especially if the potential victims may lack the abilities or resources to protect themselves.

Mental illnesses and addictions can result in serious risks to the individual: suicide, self-neglect (e.g., poor hygiene), self-harm (e.g., cutting, pulling out hair, repetitive scratching). Governmental powers to hospitalize, restrain, seclude, or treat against a person's wishes, when her behaviours are due to mental illness, are often legally set out in mental health legislation. The same legislation will specify who is legally obligated to forcibly act against the person's wishes when other people could be harmed or at risk of harm by her due to the mental health problem. If there is no actual or suspected mental health problem, then the individual would be dealt with according to applicable civil or criminal laws. Questions about the kind (physical only or psychological too?), the probability, the urgency or imminence (within the next few days or longer?), the seriousness or significance (life-threatening, disabling and/or dignity-threatening?) arise when such legislation is written or revised. While mental health legislation in most jurisdictions agrees that governmental intervention is warranted when death or serious physical harm is likely, there is disagreement as to whether other harms should be unilaterally and forcibly prevented. Similar questions arise in healthcare settings when healthcare workers, family members and the police try to decide whether to invoke their government-delegated powers.

Governmental legislation should try to strike a balance between the safety of the individual and others and the magnitude and duration of restrictions imposed upon the individual. Which rights and freedoms enjoyed by other citizens will she lose and for how long? What are the least invasive and limiting options? These questions probe whether the response to her harmful behaviour focuses on maintaining safety or on punishing undesirable behaviours.

4.4 Institutional mechanisms

Punishment is a worry for mental health facilities because their competing goals include keeping individual clients safe and keeping others safe. There are four theories of punishment: retributive theory, deterrence theory, rehabilitative theory, and restorative theory. The last three of these theories happen to resonate with various clinical paradigms. Such coherence can unintentionally link punishment with clinical interventions. It is crucial for clinicians and teams to focus on the behaviours and decisions that relate to the health problem for which the client is seeking therapeutic help. Interventions and accompanying interactions must not be punitive.

A recent judicial trend is the creation of "mental health courts" and "drug treatment courts." Their objective is to divert those who have been found guilty of violating certain laws, albeit as non-violent crimes, away from prisons and jails. The mitigating factor in this sentencing is that these people broke a particular law because of a mental illness or addiction. The fact that someone has a mental health or addiction problem does not mean that all his or her actions and choices are determined by the problem. To qualify for "medical diversion," the law-breaking actions have to be the result of the health problem; for instance, the person's judgment was impaired because he or she was intoxicated or responding to paranoid thoughts or to threatening internal voices. Accordingly, a judge decides whether the person should be diverted to an appropriate health facility to receive treatment and care for the mental health or addiction problem. Historically, judicial systems have provided no or minimal mental health and addictions treatment because punishment and control were the priorities and funding was inadequate. Focused, integrated, and sustained treatment in hospitals' programs is expected to help these individuals return to the community more quickly and not re-offend. Those who are directed to mental health and drug treatment courts usually can choose to have their cases heard in "regular court" with the possibility that if found guilty, jail, prison or probation is next. However it has been found that those who agree to be diverted into the health system may be under its auspices longer than if they had been in jail or prison. It can seem that diversion is harsher and thus less fair. This harkens back to the lack of highly effective, of easily sustained therapies or of adequate community services to justify a conditional discharge.

Therapeutic jurisprudence is a concept first coined by David Wexler, a professor of law and psychology, in a 1987 NIH conference paper (Corvette, 2000). He held that judicial systems and processes can be beneficial or harmful to those who break civil or criminal laws. Being held responsible, treated fairly, assisted in exercising rights to a fair hearing as well as others having duties to follow the impartial rule of law are considered to be psychologically and existentially affirmative of the individual as an equal member of the community. Moreover, the judicial system can help mediate injustices experienced in the public realm: "Therapeutic jurisprudence is normative. It suggests that to the extent possible, consonant with due process and justice values and goals, undesirable effects should be avoided or minimized and positive effects should be maximized" (Ibid, 103). Therapeutic jurisprudence fits with mental health courts and drug treatment courts to a degree. These court settings bring together employees of two major societal endeavours: the judiciary and healthcare. Nevertheless, caution is warranted. Various legal scholars and academics worry that these employees' roles will illegitimately merge such that role boundaries are crossed. In other words, the judicial employees will weigh in too far---beyond their knowledge and training---into the work of the healthcare employees and vice versa (Dickie, 2008; Moore, 2007; Nolan, 2003). Furthermore, benefits vary between women and men. This, in turn, warrants increased study as to different stakeholders' views about the meaning as well as the effects of these courts and their processes (Hunt et al., 2007; Moore, 2007; Shaffer et al., 2009).

Similar debates have arisen when legislatures have considered amending existing mental health laws to include community treatment orders. These orders, often called involuntary community treatment, are meant to organize a mixed set of supportive community services so that a person can leave the hospital and live safely in the community as a less restrictive option. If, however, the community providers and agencies do not fulfill their responsibilities and it is possible that the person will become unsafe as a result, then he can be forcibly re-hospitalized forthwith. At issue is how to ethically evaluate this option: solely on probable consequences (e.g., fewer urgent hospitalizations, shorter hospitalizations)? At present, not enough is known as to why community treatment orders are associated with certain positive outcomes. Are they due to the ongoing availability of comprehensive supports or is it due to the ever-present threat of the client being re-hospitalized against his will? (Burns & Dawson, 2009; Hunt et al., 2005).

Mental health and addictions settings encounter another challenge in the guise of advance directives. Advance directives have been discussed for years in the context of physical, acute care medicine. Medical advance directives permit people to designate who will be their healthcare decision proxy and/or to provide guidelines for subsequent decisions when they no longer have the capacity to decide on their own behalf. Empirical evidence shows that psychiatric advance directives, or "crisis cards" in the U.K., reduce the frequency and length of emergency hospitalizations. They also increase clinician-client trust (Srebnik & Russo, 2008; Sutherby et al., 1999). Yet discussions about psychiatric advanced directives' usefulness often ignore a critical detail: can directives be invoked *before* persons satisfy legislated criteria to be deemed incapable? Or can they be invoked only after they are assessed as lacking capacity? The "after" scenario is not too ethically or legally controversial because the directive actually constitutes client participation in the care plan and establishes relevant "prior expressed wishes" (Bogdanoski, 2009; Srebnik et al., 2005; Swanson et al., 2006). Dubbed "a Ulysses contract" after the Greek fable about Ulysses, the "before" scenario is definitely controversial. If there are legislated standards and court rulings to protect decision-making by capable citizens, then it could prove difficult, perhaps legally impossible, for citizens to waive their right to such decisional protection.

5. Why organizational context matters ethically

In the early decades of bioethics inquiry, academic and professional scrutiny and debate centred on the work of researchers using human subjects and "bedside" or "front line" practitioners. The issue that expanded this focus to include administrators, management and executives, and Board members was, I believe, the galloping costs of healthcare services that were not adequately reimbursed by governmental and private insurance plans. In the United States, Medicare's and Medicaid's decision in the 1980s to shift from reimbursing as per diagnostic Related Diagnostic Groups and to capitated managed care costs confirmed the immense impact of management on client-professional relationships. Moreover, increasing annual deficits made the *business* of healthcare an issue for everyone, from patients, practitioners, hospitals, commercial employers to governmental health ministers. All economically developed nations now experience demand exceeding healthcare supply, despite increasing budgets. Continued technological advances are typically more costly and citizens' confidence that "new" and "more" produces better health outcomes is often short-lived.

An "organization" will herein be defined as a designated group of specially trained or skilled people working towards a shared goal or purpose. As such, a rural adolescent drug counselling office consisting of three addictions workers and an office administrator constitutes an organization, as does each discrete unit within a psychiatric hospital, as does the hospital as a whole. Organizational considerations are not the concern or responsibility of only executive management; they are the responsibility of virtually all staff members.

5.1 Organizational factors

Organizational considerations in healthcare fall into four general categories, each of which warrants a brief explanation as to its relevance for ethical practice in mental health and addictions settings. One category is the ethics of the organization's mission or mandate. The purpose of an organization, irrespective of whether it has been formally and explicitly described or it is implicit in its regular activities, establishes to whom the organization is responsible and accountable and for what… and to whom it is not responsible. More simply put, a mandate sets out the groups of people to whom the organization must respond with "Yes, we can help you" and to whom it can respond legitimately with "You will have to look elsewhere for assistance." In contemporary healthcare, healthcare organizations have often developed a set of values to guide how their mission and strategic goals are accomplished. A point in this chapter's introduction bears repeating here: some values are intrinsically ethical (e.g., being trustworthy, relieving suffering). Other values may be instrumentally ethical (i.e., financial stewardship so as to maximize number of clients served).

A second category is the ethics of how a healthcare organization is governed: what should be the guiding operational standards and according to whom? Governance will be both internal and external. Examples of external governance include accreditation standards, employment and occupational health regulations, applicable government legislation, funding regulations, professional Colleges' codes of practice, and the organization's Board of Trustees/Directors. Examples of internal governance include negotiated labour contracts, a code of employee conduct, quality-safety committee, any document that details patient rights as well as the largest and most endemic "repository" of internal governance, written policies and procedures.

Another general organizational ethics category for healthcare settings is the ethics of resource acquisition, allocation, and disposal. Here, "resources" applies not just to money, but also to staff, beds, counselling sessions, equipment, physical space, and professionals' time. How resources are obtained is ethically important, as evidenced by debates about seeking funds from pharmaceutical and gaming corporations or about recruiting nurses and professionals from countries sorely lacking in qualified personnel. Allocation of resources, as mentioned earlier, is the most well known organizational ethics issue in health care: how to allocate resources fairly, even if there is just "soft" scarcity, is challenging and often is informed only by an implicit utilitarian calculus. Prioritizing access to and provision of in-patient or out-patient services occurs routinely and includes wide-ranging decisions such as which medications to include or exclude from a hospital formulary, how to respond to "VIP requests" for access, and how many times a hospitalized client or his substitute decision maker can decline a community bed without consequence. Resource "disposal" first came to attention vis-à-vis discussions about the environmental impact of what was being discarded by tertiary, acute care hospitals. Yet closing or reducing services can mean staff layoffs and reduced hours. Refreshing all computer hardware can mean deciding whether to donate the replaced computers to a remote school or a community centre serving people living with addictions problems. "Disposal" decisions involve ethics-related values such as who will be harmed versus benefited, who should help identify alternatives and applicable rationales, and who is responsible for making the final decision.

The last category is the ethics of an organization's culture and climate. Understanding what culture and climate are and their impact has been a favoured topic in business ethics and business literature for some time. Culture is reflected in what is considered acceptable versus unacceptable behaviour and interactions. It is so ingrained and presumed to be "right" that it does not need to be written anywhere. Culture will include norms for how hard staff should work, what counts as humour, what questions can and cannot be asked out loud, and how much is decided by committees versus individuals. Climate is a metaphoric word to capture the organization's current mood: is it optimistic, such that trying something new without administrative permission is a safe thing to do? Or is it suspicious, such that "not rocking the boat" is well advised? Or is it celebratory such that being a little less productive for awhile is acceptable?

In virtually all ethics related questions involving clients, organizational considerations will implicitly or explicitly impact their treatment, care, and interactions with co-clients, staff, family members, and outside parties. In some instances, staff responses will be ethically weaker or stronger because of these considerations. Some everyday examples include practices and policies about smoking restrictions, searching clients' belongings, hospitalized clients' intimate and sexual behaviours, clients' use of illegal substances during the therapy period, staff responses when clients may be driving impaired, staff obligations or lack thereof if a pregnant client uses illegal substances, and so on. Policies and practices must balance competing, often conflicting, interests and responsibilities. As noted by Winkler (2005), depending on how policies are developed and implemented, they can minimize the power and resource imbalances among staff as well as between clients and staff. Or they can exacerbate them. As memorably explained in Skorpen et al.'s (2008) article about smoking rooms in a psychiatric facility, clients can try to find ways to regain power and equal status. On a separate but related point, safety initiatives will be ethically grounded. However, safety can become the "sun" that blocks out all other considerations, or "a trump card" that silences all other interests and voices. Depending on a healthcare facility's culture and climate, it may be politically unwise to suggest that safety measures are causing more burdens and disadvantages than anticipated.

Busy clinics and hospitals may operate unintentionally in ways that traumatize or re-traumatize clients. Many people who develop a mental health or addiction problem have experienced serious trauma, be it physical, emotional, and/or psychological abuse. If a medical office or health clinic's practices are impersonal, coercive, or disrespectful, the person may find them even more distressful and stressful because her past experiences of being silenced, pressured, or shamed are remembered and reinforced. Moreover programs and units may operate with such allegiance to "the rules" that professional judgement and integrity fade. Having integrity requires some modicum of inner struggle, according to scholar Stephen Carter (1996). In other words, having integrity is praiseworthy *because* it is hard to achieve. Therefore if healthcare workers' motives for acting as they do come from "following the rules," then they might be commended as being capable rule followers, but this is divorced from being professional or having integrity. As noted in the introduction, reasons for acting may not be based on ethics-related values, but instead on other considerations such as self-interest, convenience, power, or fatigue.

5.2 Forensic programs and services

The ethical challenges and complexities of forensic healthcare programs and settings are numerous and significant, as reflected throughout this chapter. In the case of forensic services, care is needed to avoid unintentional "creep" of the police and prison system into the therapeutic system. Language is an obvious marker of such ingress: clients or patients have privileges that they can lose, regain, and exercise. Yet the word "privileges" evokes imperialism and parentalism because privileges are granted by one party to another. If an empowering or strengths-based approach is adopted instead, clinicians could refer to a client's "responsibilities" or "actions" as set out in the court or review board order. There would be consequences, positive and negative, if she fulfills or does not fulfill her responsibilities, rather than the moralizing or infant-alizing rhetoric of "consequences to reward good behaviour." To help balance the power relations more equitably, her clinical team and the program management would also have various responsibilities to fulfill. Another example is contraband, wherein clients are prohibited from having certain qualifying items with them in the hospital. But "contraband" is a familiar police and drug enforcement word related to smuggling. It does not belong in a healing environment (recall that the person was diverted *from* the prison or jail system). Alternative wording could be "unsafe items" or "prohibited items," which are accurate descriptions but far less polarizing. Ethics texts written for psychologists and psychiatrists usually include a chapter on ethically defensible ways to formally assess a person for court such that the person does not mistakenly presume the clinician has her best interests in mind. As noted above, health workers may struggle to maintain the appropriate balance between offering therapy and following a court's legitimate demands. It is essential for programs to proactively and openly examine their routine practices. These forums will help support workers to deal with the to-be-expected moral distress of meeting competing commitments (Austin, 2001; Morse, 2008; Pouncey & Lukens, 2010). Moreover understanding clients' actual experiences of these situations, rather than just working from assumptions, is important because the significant power differential between clinician and client can progressively erode professional commitments.

6. Why systemic factors matter ethically

Since moving from a large tertiary, acute care hospital to working at a large mental health and addictions hospital, systemic factors have figured prominently in my ethical analyses and recommendations. Like Sokol, I gradually became aware of these factors' impact on the daily lives of clients, families, and healthcare workers alike as I listened to more and more personal stories: someone who can only afford substandard housing and worries bedbugs will soon infiltrate their belongings, a recreational therapist frustrated that clients are not welcome at a community gym, and rural parents whose employer-paid insurance plan caps psychotherapy for their behaviourally aggressive child at ten sessions per year. Systemic factors are implicit in a community or society's ongoing activities that occur just outside the walls of a private practice, clinic, or hospital. Three kinds of factors are particularly relevant to defensibly determining normative responses or, in other words, "what should happen." Moreover these factors ground any health and healthcare decision in the reality of a particular society or community. Sidestepping these factors in ethics-related analyses can result in ineffective responses or assigning responsibilities disproportionately.

6.1 Stigma

The first ethically weighty factor is stigma. There are many definitions of stigma, but Jo Phelan and Bruce Link (2001) offer a nuanced characterization. They suggest that it has four components, which appropriately captures its complexity: (1) human differences are identified and labelled, (2) these differences are linked to negative qualities, (3) those who are different become "Them" as separate from "Us", and (4) the person's or group's social status declines and unfair discrimination occurs. Those who make up society's majority, captive to the seeming truth of "bell curve statistics," commonly presume that what is common constitutes what is "normal" and what is uncommon constitutes what is not just rare, but also what is morally abnormal. As described by historical accounts of societies' treatment of those whose thinking was unusual, this treatment has traditionally been fear-based and repressive. Furthermore, if people's thoughts were accompanied by behaviours and appearances that violated social etiquette and norms, the collective responses included dismissive marginalization, controlled quarantine, or forced treatment. Historically, mainly charitable or faith-based institutions endeavoured to care for and about people with mental illnesses until the past fifty years or so in North America and Europe. Yet stigma remains a contemporary problem. For example, based on its 2006 Senate report on mental illnesses and addictions and available services, *Out of the Shadows at Last*, Canada's Mental Health Commission launched "Opening Minds," a *ten*-year anti-stigma/anti-discrimination initiative.

Social or communal stigmatization and discrimination----related to ethics concepts of de-humanization and injustice----help explain why most people are initially reluctant to seek psychiatric and psychological testing because of the enduring harms of being labelled as having a mental health or addictions problem. Families, too, delay seeking information and help from clinicians and programs, often relying primarily on the Internet's anonymity and non-judgemental-ness. Keeping health problems secret limits access as well as limits offers of needed, physical, psychological, relational, educational, and economic support. Yet stigma and discrimination go beyond the general public's response to those living with a mental health or addiction problem. Studies have also revealed that many mental health and addictions workers unconsciously and consciously stigmatize and discriminate against their own clients despite their day-to-day interactions with them (Flanagan et al., 2009; Liggins & Hatcher, 2005; Ross, 2009; Schulze, 2007). There is also evidence that mental health and addiction workers themselves are stigmatized by working in this field of healthcare (Gouthro, 2010; Halter, 2008; Stuhlmiller, 2005).

Discrimination of individuals with mental health and addictions problems can be more subtle, but can be just as unfair. It is important to examine whether double standards are being presumed or relied upon. Clinicians and teams may want to restrict client activities that would be permitted in general society. For example, a residential program may decide to permit residents to engage in consensual, non-exploitative intimate behaviours in their private rooms, but expect these behaviours to reflect "highly responsible" or "meaningful" activity. Or the program may have a search policy that presumes residents to be more dangerous and more devious than has been actually experienced. Media stories and mainstream television and movie companies sensationalize rare disorders and behaviours as well as behaviours that result in criminal charges or convictions. For instance, programs and healthcare workers' attention can be disproportionately directed to people's use of illegal drugs compared to their tobacco and alcohol use. Yet smoking and drinking alcohol cause more death and serious co-morbidities than marijuana, or even heroin.

Language is slow to change, too. Someone in treatment for, say, cocaine addiction is said to "test dirty" on a urine drug screen (Radcliffe & Stevens, 2008; Rose et al., 2005). Urine screens for people with diabetes, however, are described as "testing positive" or "negative.". As "addicts," "schizophrenics" or "sex offenders," people are reduced to a particular illness or behavioural category. There has been a move within the addictions field to talk about substance dependence, misuse, and abuse… rather than always about addictions. Hofman et al's 2003 study of inner city women who were IV-drug users and used outreach health services far less than male IV-drug users in the same area revealed the women's ongoing efforts to fulfill familial and communal responsibilities plus retain a sense of respectability. The criticism of healthcare workers' continued use of the demeaning and paternalistic terms "compliance" and "non-compliance" is about stigma as well (Acosta et al., 2009; Bissella et al., 2004; Proulx et al., 2007; Stewart & DeMarco, 2010). Because of stigma, discrimination, negative side effects, and human nature, it should not surprise us that people do not follow prescribed regimens at the high level of "compliance" needed. As noted by a systems and client advocate, those receiving health services do not set a personal goal of "being more compliant" with their treatment (Jennifer Chambers, 2010; personal communications). Instead, they set more meaningful goals such as getting sustainable employment, feeling well enough to help with a son's homework, or having more faith in one's hard-won wisdom.

6.2 Social determinants of health

Being healthy does not rely solely on physiology, genetics, and lifestyle choices. Social and cultural factors also have significant impact (Lauder et al., 2007). While the World Health Organization (2003) identifies several social determinants, three are of particular ethical import for mental health and addictions contexts: housing, unemployment and poverty, and social isolation. The percentage of people who are homeless and have a mental illness, while difficult to accurately determine, is estimated to range from 20% to up to 50% in various studies of Canadian, U.K. and American cities (Hwang, 2001; Meltzer, 2008; National Coalition for the Homeless, 2009; Neale, 2008; Senate Standing Committee, 2006). The relationship between unstable and inadequate housing and mental illness and addictions is considered to be bi-directional. In other words, sub-standard housing contributes to onset or relapse just as mental illness and addictions contribute to loss of adequate and reliable housing. Reflective of continued discrimination, "NIMBY" or "not in my back yard" is a common community response, opposing governmental or private agency housing initiatives for people with persistent health concerns, such as mental illnesses and addictions.

People with mental health and addictions problems are at increased risk of living in poverty (Canadian Mental Health Association, 2007; Hudson, 2005; Wilton, 2004). Schizophrenia, for instance, usually manifests in late adolescence or young adulthood, which means educational efforts are disrupted. Lack of post-secondary education usually results in being less competitive in the job market. Stigma means that finding suitable employment is more difficult---even though many countries have legislation prohibiting discrimination based on health conditions---and once employed, people must often be diligent to keep their mental health or addictions history secret. Governments may offer financial assistance to those unable to work due to a physical or mental disability, but the amount of support typically provides for a low standard of living.

Psychiatric hospitals were once known as "asylums" because they were considered safe havens from the uncertainties and rigors of daily life. But too many became immense institutions of sturdy walls and high fences in which people with mental health problems lived out their lives separated from the community. Exclusion is anathema to human health and well-being. Moreover, some mental illnesses, such as autism, paranoia, and personality disorders, involve reduced abilities to understand or trust other people and this, in turn, undermines relationship-building. Add public prejudice and the consequences for many people with mental health problems are isolation and marginalization (Baum et al., 2010; Elisha et al., 2006; Morgan et al., 2008 and 2007; Smith & Hirdes 2009).

6.3 Health and social systems writ large

The third systemic factor that is ethically noteworthy is our social and health systems. Three issues help illustrate the tangible impact of these systems on the therapies available and the recovery realized. First, ethically worrisome conflicts of interest can exist. When a government sells alcohol and operates gambling venues (e.g., casinos, lotteries), this runs counter to its public health mandate (Andresen, 2006; Livingstone & Adams, 2011; Walker & Jackson; 2011). Even if a government only regulates commercial sales of these items and activities, their coffers receive immense sums of money from luxury taxes on alcohol, gambling, and cigarettes. As evidenced by the "Big Tobacco Settlement" in the United States, only a few of the 48 states in the class action suit directed a substantial part of their proportion of the $235 billion settlement to smoking prevention and treatment. The other states assigned their settlement portion to deficit reduction, infrastructure needs, and more general uses (Johnson, 2004).

Another systemic issue is the historic and continued unfair insurance coverage or reimbursement for non-physician and non-hospital therapies. For instance, Canadian provincial and territorial governments' health insurance plans tend to not reimburse psychotherapies or alternative treatments provided by non-physicians in the community, but do reimburse physician-provided/prescribed and/or hospital-based treatments. In most cases, psychologist/therapist and psychological measures are either paid by employer insurance plans or out-of-pocket (Parker & Burke, 2005). These plans usually cap their coverage at low levels. In fact, the U.S. Congress passed the Mental Health Parity and Addiction Equity Act in 2008 to help address this inequity by requiring federal health plans to reimburse mental health services on par with medical health services.

Systemic considerations contribute to "revolving door situations," which are usually and unfairly identified as "revolving door patients." These situations centre on health gains, made by someone while receiving the intensive and publicly provided services in a hospital, dissipating quickly once he returns to the community which may lack certain services, or have insufficient services, or have services that are neither easily understood nor effective. Continuity of care and comprehensiveness of services falter. As a result, he soon requires re-hospitalization to receive more intensive and comprehensive therapies. Returning to home may mean that the benefits prove unsustainable and re-hospitalization is likely. This repetitive cycle is particularly concerning if the illness is such that it is not physiologically possible to return fully to the pre-crisis levels of functioning. Health system reform and social system reform appear on most countries' election platforms, but reform is difficult to achieve given the programs' immense complexity and the perpetual expectation of increased funding.

7. Conclusion

7.1 Cases revisited

How can these various recommendations and cautions deepen and refine our understanding of the cases at the opening of this chapter and shift our responses from what is minimally ethical to what is optimally ethical?

Case 1: First, the nurse should verify what the applicable legislation states in terms of which, if any, healthcare professional is responsible for reporting what, to whom, and based on what evidence. If the legislation does assign responsibility, is it to just a physician or to any healthcare worker who has direct contact with a client? If to a physician only, is the nurse *legally* expected to notify the physician? Is the responsibility framed as obligatory or permissible? In terms of evidence, is it in the form of a professional assessment or a mere belief or opinion? Answers to such questions should guide the nurse in terms of what she says to the physician and what she and/or the physician say to Sergei.

Even if there is no applicable legislation, this remains a possible *health* concern that the physician should broach supportively with him. Alcohol dependence rates are highest in Russia, therefore it is more likely that he, too, has a substance use problem, or at the very least, may be experiencing some personal challenges for which he is misusing alcohol to cope. If the physician and/or nurse conclude they do have a legal duty to report, it remains their decision as to whether they actually will contact the Ministry. They may decide instead to talk first with Sergei, learn more about his drinking pattern and motivations, and inform

him of their legal obligation to report. In so doing, they are weighing the likely consequences to Sergei, his family members (who may be in the car when he is impaired), and the general public. They may also believe openness and support will help preserve their therapeutic relationship with him and increase the likelihood that if he is misusing alcohol, he will pursue treatment and/or counselling. If the clinicians report Sergei to the Ministry and the Ministry decides to revoke his licence, they should be willing to support---if they have relevant corroborating information regarding his successful efforts to control the medical condition that resulted in dangerous driving---a license re-application in the future.
Case 2: A team member should find out exactly what the Mental Health Act states. It is careless and unprofessional to rely on unfounded assumptions and beliefs. The harmfulness of sexually transmitted diseases (STDs) is subject to debate. For instance, some STDs are not reportable under any provincial or state public health regulation, some are reportable only in certain jurisdictions, and some STDs are reportable in every jurisdiction. Moreover, is involuntary hospitalization the least restrictive preventive measure? The team may be illegitimately presuming that Ana Li herself considers pregnancy or an STD something to prevent. Paternalism needs to be tempered as do any moral judgments about "unwed mothers," "inadequate mothering," or promiscuity. It is unclear whether Ana-Li lacks the capacity to be making decisions about measures to reduce the likelihood of STDs, pregnancy, or about engaging in sexual activity. Hypersexuality alone does not imply incapacity. The team must share their concerns with Ana-Li and do so in a sensitive and mature way. It should not be assumed that all team members are experienced and skilled enough to talk about sexuality and intimacy.

If, however, she is found to lack the capacity to make decisions about such preventive measures, the team should turn to her mother to make the related medical decisions. The team will need to be more skilful in their discussions with Ana Li's mother so that it will be the client's values that are respected. It is to be expected that parents and young adults will differ about the meaning and risks of intimate activity and pregnancy. Admittedly single parenthood tends to be difficult financially and otherwise, but this is often due to societal constraints, rather than the individual's apathy. Diligence is needed to not lapse into double standards wherein most parents are given considerable latitude yet those with mental health problems must reach a far higher standard. It would not be surprising if a team member suggests early notification of a local child protection agency because of the possibility that Ana-Li could become pregnant and unable to care for a child. However this is a "rush to judgment" and may reflect prejudice and disrespect. Moreover, once the call to the agency is made, it cannot be "unmade" and Ana-Li's name may be recorded in its system indefinitely. This could be stigmatizing and may negatively affect her in the future.

Case 3: The program clients' health should improve and be sustained longer by having peer workers' support and advice and by having staff understand how their homes (or more often, "housing") contribute to or erode their well-being. Team members should benefit professionally as well, because peer workers' knowledge can help counter over-reliance on the medical model and home visits help members identify and tailor services better to clients' circumstances and thus be more effective. But clinical considerations---which relate to ethics because they are about meaningful benefits for those involved---do not exhaust this case. A peer support worker can be a very special role: for instance, it may be designed such that workers do not "do" therapy or provide treatment. Nor do they fill in for absent family or friends, helping to occupy clients' free time. Instead, peer support workers have their own expertise and ways to support clients in being as healthy as they wish. Team members may unintentionally induce peer support workers to take on their work and thereby violate role boundaries. Peer workers themselves may be attracted unconsciously to the seemingly greater authority of the professionals, especially if the workers work side-by-side with the clinic or hospital staff. These are organizational considerations.

Ethically, power, authority, and voice are involved here which means that client trust of the team and workers is at stake, just as is the trust between the team and the workers. The initiative about home visits is ethically complex because some clients may prefer to keep their homes private, away from the team's "medical gaze." Other clients, however, may appreciate home visits because of the convenience, plus it may help equalize the power in their relationship with team members. Team members may not appreciate this implicit loss of power. And if client lives in a risky area of town, team members may be reluctant to visit alone, but program resources may be heavily strained if staff make home visits in pairs. Nonetheless, equity of access to healthcare services demands proportional efforts (greater efforts if access is harder) to reach those living in inhospitable areas due to poverty resulting from having a serious mental illness or addiction, compared to efforts to reach those living in safer areas. Neither initiative should be unilaterally imposed on clients, despite how clinically sensible the initiatives seem. The director, managers, and leads should seek input from a representative group of clients to ensure that both initiatives fit clients' circumstances and needs well. Furthermore, since the director is new to the program, he must act in trustworthy ways in the hope that all his staff will genuinely commit to his overarching vision, of which the two initiatives are representative.

Case 4: It may not be ethically sufficient for someone with good oratory skills to speak on behalf of Jane. Given the historical treatment of individuals with mental health problems, providing them opportunities to use their own "voice" can signal respect and a better equalization of power. Moreover, the team should not assume that their therapeutic relationship with Jane is more important than her relationship with the lawyer. Exercising one's legal options and participating in the judicial system are valuable citizenship rights. The team may also be presuming incorrectly that the lawyer did not explain to Jane the possible pros and cons of her testifying and how the Board would likely interpret her remarks. Moreover, Jane may have decided that the benefits of speaking---to affirm her courage to "stand before" those who will judge her case and to have them listen to her---outweigh the possible risks. Team members may be ascribing to an erroneous stereotype wherein Legal Aid lawyers are believed to be less skilled than Crown attorneys and corporate lawyers. At the outset of Jane's hospitalization, the team should have discussed with her what their responsibilities are to her, to the Review Board, and to her lawyer, and any competing, possibly conflicting, commitments. Leaving such conversations until just before a Board hearing is inappropriate. The team should encourage Jane to see them and her lawyer as available resources to her to help her return to the community, but refrain from *telling* her what she should do to receive a conditional release.

Case 5: Is Omar revoking his consent when he says he does not want to go to the specialist? If "yes" but the team ignores the revocation because debridement is "clearly in his best interests" and his ulcers are debrided, this would constitute assault. What if the team concludes that at the time he says he does not want to go, he lacks the capacity to decide against debridement? Does his prior agreement when he had capacity still apply? This situation illustrates the telling difference between consent to treatment---a decisional activity---and cooperation with treatment---a physical and behavioural activity. Trying to take him to the specialist's office may result in an escalating situation of angry words, raised voices, threatening statements and then a "code" has to be called. This may damage the therapeutic relationship such that when Omar regains capacity, he may decide that returning to his home as quickly as possible is his best immediate option. Furthermore, Omar's refusal to go to the hospital may reflect many people's common reluctance and vacillation about seeing medical practitioners and therapists. Understanding clients' statements and behaviours should not be reduced just to medical considerations (i.e., non-compliance) or legal considerations (i.e., lacking capacity). Rather, it is crucial to see clients first as everyday people with many similar habits, preferences, and interests as everyone else. In other words, Omar's wish to not go to the specialist may be the response of most people who must go to big hospitals or have non-healing ulcers debrided. Those who are not in a hospital would just phone the specialist's office and ask for a later appointment. But Omar is in the hospital. The clinical team are now involved and may be unknowingly making it *their* care plan, rather than *his* care plan.

Case 6: Money can compromise organizational and personal integrity and reputation alike. The representatives should generate a variety of ideas to cover the costs without sacrificing the number who will attend or who can attend. The considerable profits of pharmaceutical and alcohol businesses means they have ready resources to increase their name recognition and brand loyalty. The agency representatives should find out what are the kinds of restrictions or limits academic healthcare institutions---which have long worried about conflicts of interest, unbalanced content, and reduced credibility---have instituted in terms of financial support from commercial enterprises and use these as guidelines. Moreover, it is worthwhile investigating whether the industries have set their own detailed guidelines for donations. As illustrated by the Code of Ethical Practices of Canadian research-based pharmaceutical companies (Rx&D, 2010), industries may want to avoid perceptions of excess and undue influence in order to protect their corporate reputation. In terms of the lottery, will it increase attendance enough to cover the spa's cost? Can the lottery be replaced by a draw wherein all registrants receive just one ticket? If the spa weekend is of modest value, it is unlikely to lure those with gambling problems. And much time will pass between registration and the draw, which means immediate gratification from winning, a risk factor of problem gambling, is almost impossible.

Case 7: Keeping secrets is risky, whether the secret-holder is the person with the health problem, a family member, or a clinician. In the short-term, the benefits of secrets may outweigh harms. Nonetheless, it can become more and more difficult to keep them. The harm of nondisclosure may increase as time passes. The "right time" to break the silence about the secret may never appear, but Edward's health problem is long-term. Moreover, what explains his continued visits to the physician? And what explains the seeming inconsistency between taking the renewed prescriptions and yet not having them filled? Qualitative studies have revealed that people have sound reasons for what appears initially to be noncompliance with the recommended treatment.

In terms of Sandra and her partner, they should not be expected to keep their home open to Edward indefinitely. Women continue to fulfill most of the demands of family and home life in most societies, a continued sign of societal discrimination. It is thus inappropriate for the physician to presume that Sandra and her partner still want to or should have Edward reside with them. To address this quandary ethically, the physician should let Sandra know that it is not, and was not, legally or ethically appropriate for him to take advantage of the secret administration of the prescription medication. He can suggest that Sandra explain to Edward what she has done and why and be supportive if she is worried that Edward will react in a threatening or unsafe way. The physician should invite Edward to his office to discuss what has happened, why and provide information and resources to help Edward remain as healthy as he wishes. In the spirit of not abandoning his patient and since it is possible that the physician-patient relationship will be broken, the physician should be prepared to offer Edward the names of other clinicians with whom he can find therapeutic support and access medical treatments.

7.2 Wrap-up

In summary, people and their communities are complex. Problems with our cognitive and emotional abilities have profound effects. Understanding and defining human cognition and emotions and their interconnections continues to evolve in psychiatry, psychology, neurology, and neuroscience. Moreover, recent research and clinical advances in neurology and neuroscience have led to the emergence of neuroethics, the newest field within bioethics and one focused on the human brain and nervous system. In a sense, science and what is traditionally known as the medical complex have - rightly or wrongly - not yet assumed in relation to mental health and addictions the authoritative position they have in physical medicine and acute care settings.

Foundational ethical commitments and values remain relevant: for instance, the person's own wisdom and perspective, the community's obligations to all its members, the duties and limits of the state's intervention in individual and familial lives, a holistic view of factors contributing to individual and group well-being, and the immense, lasting harms of discrimination and stigma. Therefore, ethical understanding, engagement, and assistance for people's mental health and addiction problems, requires in-depth and broad analyses, multi-faceted and integrated responses, "the long view" and abiding commitment, non-replication of past power imbalances and moralization, and a defensible role or place for law and legislation.

8. References

Acosta, F, Bosch, E, Sarmiento, G, Juanes, N, Caballero-Hidalgo, A & Mayans, T. (2009). Evaluation of Noncompliance in Schizophrenia Patients Using Electronic Monitoring (MEMS) and its Relationship to Sociodemographic, Clinical and Psychopathological Variables. *Schizophrenia Research*, Vol. 107, Nos. 2-3 (February 2009), pp. 213-7, ISSN 0920-9964.

Amiel, J, Mangurian, C, Ganguli, R & Newcomer, J. (2008). Addressing Cardiometabolic Risk During Treatment with Antipsychotic Medications. *Current Opinion in Psychiatry*, Vol. 21, No. 6 (November 2008), pp. 613-8, ISSN 0951-7367.

Andresen, M. (2006). Governments' Conflict of Interest in Treating Problem Gamblers. *CMAJ*, Vol. 175, No. 10 (November 2006), pp. 1191, ISSN 1488-2329. Aristotle. (2009). *Nicomachean Ethics*, World Classics Library, ISBN 019283407X, Des Moines

Austin, W. (2001). Relational Ethics in Forensic Psychiatric Settings. *Journal of Psychosocial Nursing & Mental Health Services*, Vol. 39, No. 9 (September 2001), pp. 12-7, ISSN 0279-3695.

Banzato, C. (2004). Classification in Psychiatry: the move towards ICD-11 and DSM-V. *Current Opinion in Psychiatry*, Vol. 17, No. 6 (November 2004), pp. 497-501, ISSN 0951-7367.

Baum, F, Newman, L, Biedrzycki, K & Patterson, J. (2010). Can a Regional Government's Social Inclusion Initiative Contribute to the Quest for Health Equity? *Health Promotion International*, Vol. 25, No. 4 (December 2010), pp. 474-82, ISSN 0957-4824.

Bissella, P, May, C & Noyce, P. (2004). From Compliance to Concordance: barriers to accomplishing a re-framed model of health care interactions. *Social Science & Medicine*, Vol. 58, No. 4 (February 2004), pp. 851–62, ISSN 0277-9536.

Bogdanoski, T. (2009). Psychiatric Advance Directives: the new frontier in mental health law reform in Australia? *Journal of Law & Medicine*, Vol. 16, No. 5 (May 2009), pp. 891-904, ISSN 1320-159X.

Burns, T & Dawson, J. (2009). Community Treatment Orders: how ethical without experimental evidence? *Psychological Medicine*, Vol. 39, No. 10 (October 2009), pp. 1583-6, ISSN 0033-2917.

Canadian Mental Health Association. (2007). *Poverty and Mental Illness*. Retrieved from www.ontario.cmha.ca/backgrounders.asp?cID=25341.

Carter, S. (1996). *Integrity*. HarperPerennial, ISBN 9780060928070, New York.

Cleveland, M, Feinberg, M & Greenberg, M. (2010). Protective Families in High- and Low-Risk Environments: implications for adolescent substance use. *Journal of Youth & Adolescence*, Vol. 39, No. 2 (February 2010), pp. 114-26, ISSN 0047-2891.

Collier, R. (2010). DSM Revision Surrounded by Controversy. *CMAJ*, Vol. 182, No. 1 (January 2010), pp. 16-7, ISSN 1488-2329.

Corvette, B. (2000). Therapeutic Jurisprudence. *Sociological Practice*, Vol. 2, No. 2 (June 2000), pp. 127-32, ISSN 1522-3442.

Dickie, I. (2008). Ethical Dilemmas, Forensic Psychology, and Therapeutic Jurisprudence. *Thomas Jefferson Law Review*, Vol. 30, No. 2 (Spring 2008), pp. 455-61, ISSN 1090-5278.

Elisha, D, Castle, D & Hocking, B. (2006). Reducing Social Isolation in People with Mental Illness: the role of the psychiatrist. *Australasian Psychiatry*, Vol. 14, No. 3 (September 2006), pp. 281-4, ISSN 1039-8562.

Finney, J & Moos, R. (2006). Matching Clients' Treatment Goals with Treatment Oriented Towards Abstinence, Moderation or Harm Reduction. *Addiction*, Vol. 101, No. 11 (November 2006), pp. 1540-2, ISSN 0968-7610.

Flanagan, E, Miller, R & Davidson, L. (2009). "Unfortunately, We Treat the Chart:" sources of stigma in mental health settings. *Psychiatric Quarterly*, Vol. 80, No. 1 (March 2009), pp. 55-64, ISSN 1573-6709.

Foucault, M. (1988). *Madness and Civilization: a history of insanity in the age of reason*. Random House, ISBN 067972110X, New York. Frank, A. (2004). Ethics as Process and Practice. *Internal Medicine Journal*, Vol. 34, No. 6 (June

Futterman, R, Lorente, M & Silverman, S. (2004). Integrating Harm Reduction and Abstinence-Based Substance Abuse Treatment in the Public Sector. *Substance Abuse*, Vol. 25, No. 1 (March 2004), pp. 3-7, ISSN 0889-7077.

Gagne, C, White, W & Anthony, W. (2007). Recovery: a common vision for the fields of mental health and addictions. *Psychiatric Rehabilitation Journal*, Vol. 31, No. 1 (Summer 2007), pp. 32-7, ISSN 1095-158X.

Gouthro, T. (2009). Recognizing and Addressing the Stigma Associated with Mental Health Nursing: a critical perspective. *Issues in Mental Health Nursing,* Vol. 30, No. 11 (November 2009), pp. 669-76, ISSN 1061-2840.

Halter, M. (2008). Perceived Characteristics of Psychiatric Nurses: stigma by association. *Archives of Psychiatric Nursing,* Vol. 22, No. 1 (February 2008), pp. 20-6, ISSN 0883-9417.

Helzer, J, Bucholz, K & Gossop, M. (2007). A Dimensional Option for the Diagnosis of Substance Dependence in DSM-V. *International Journal of Methods in Psychiatric Research,* Vol.16, No. S1 (June 2007), pp. S24-33, ISSN 1557-0657.

Hilfiker, D. (1992). The Case. Clint Wooder. *Second Opinion,* vol. 18, no. 2 (October 1992), pp. 42-53, ISSN 0890-1570.

Hofman, N, Strenski, T, Marshall, P & Heimer, R. (2003). Maintaining Respectability and Responsibility: gendered labor patterns among women injection drug users. *Health Care for Women International,* Vol. 24, No. 9 (November 2003), pp. 794–807, ISSN 0739-9332.

Holland, M. (1998). Touching the Weights: moral perception and attention. *International Philosophical Quarterly,* Vol. 38, No. 3 (September 1998), pp. 299-312, ISSN 0019-0365.

Hudson, C. (2005). Socioeconomic Status and Mental Illness: tests of the social causation and selection hypotheses. *American Journal of Orthopsychiatry,* Vol. 75, No. 1, (January 2005), pp. 3–18, ISSN 1939-0025.

Hunt, A, da Silva, A, Lurie, S & Goldbloom, D. (2007). Community Treatment Orders in Toronto: the emerging data. *Canadian Journal of Psychiatry,* Vol. 52, No. 10 (October 2007), pp. 647-56, ISSN 0706-7437.

Hwang, S. (2001) Homelessness and Health. *CMAJ,* Vol. 164, No. 2, (January 2001), pp. 229-33, ISSN 1488-2329.

Ivanova, M & Israel, A. (2006). Family Stability as a Protective Factor Against Psychopathology for Urban Children Receiving Psychological Services. *Journal of Clinical Child & Adolescent Psychology,* Vol. 35, No. 4 (December 2006), pp. 564-70, ISSN 1537-4416.

Johnson, C. (2004). The State of the Tobacco Settlement: are settlement funds being used to finance state government budget deficits? A research note. *Public Budgeting & Finance,* Vol. 24, No. 1 (March 2004), pp. 113-25, ISSN 0275-1100.

Kingdon, D & Nicholl, J. (2006). Mental Health Research Continues to be Underfunded. *BMJ,* Vol. 332, No. 7556 (June 2006), pp. 1510, ISSN 0959-8138.

Knesper, D. (2007). My Favorite Tips for Engaging the Difficult Patient on Consultation-Liaison Psychiatry Services. *Psychiatric Clinics of North America,* Vol. 30, No. 2 (June

Korol, S. (2008). Familial and Social Support as Protective Factors Against the Development of Dissociative Identity Disorder. *Journal of Trauma & Dissociation,* Vol. 9, No. 2, pp. 249-67, ISSN 1529-9732.

Kraemer, H. (2007). DSM Categories and Dimensions in Clinical and Research Contexts. *International Journal of Methods in Psychiatric Research,* Vol.16, No. S1 (June 2007), pp. S8-S15, ISSN 1557-0657.

Lauder, W, Kroll, T & Jones, M. (2007). Social Determinants of Mental Health: the missing dimensions of mental health nursing? *Journal of Psychiatric & Mental Health Nursing,* Vol. 14, No. 7 (October 2007), pp. 661-9, ISSN 1351-0126.

Lauro, L, Bass, A, Goldsmith, L, Kaplan, J, Katz, G & Schaye. S. (2003). Psychoanalytic Supervision of the Difficult Patient. *Psychoanalytic Quarterly*, Vol. 72, No. 2 (April 2003), pp. 403-38, ISSN 0033-2828.

Liggins, J & Hatcher, S. (2005). Stigma toward the Mentally Ill in the General Hospital: a qualitative study. *General Hospital Psychiatry*, Vol. 27, No. 5 (September 2005), pp. 359-64, ISSN 0163-8343.

Link, B & Phelan J. (2001). Conceptualizing Stigma. *Annual Review of Sociology*, Vol. 27, No. 1 (2001), pp. 363-85, ISSN 0360-0572.

Livingstone, C & Adams, P. (2011). Harm Promotion: observations on the symbiosis between government and private industries in Australasia for the development of highly accessible gambling markets. *Addiction*, Vol. 106, No. 1 (January 2011), pp. 3–8, ISSN 1074-3529.

Lowe, T & Lubos, E. (2008). Effectiveness of Weight Management Interventions for People with Serious Mental Illness Who Receive Treatment with Atypical Antipsychotic Medications. A literature review. *Journal of Psychiatric & Mental Health Nursing*, Vol. 15, No. 10 (December 2008), pp. 857-63, ISSN 1351-0126.

MacIntyre, A. (2007). *After Virtue: a study in moral theory*, third edition, University of Notre Dame Press, ISBN 9780268035044, Notre Dame.

Meltzer, H. (2008) State-of-Science Review: SR-B6 The Mental Ill-Health of Homeless People for *Mental Capital and Wellbeing: Making the most of ourselves in the 21st century*. Retrieved from www.bis.gov.uk/assets/bispartners/foresight/docs/mental-capital/sr-b6_mcw.pdf.

Miller, W. (2008). The Ethics of Harm Reduction, In *The Book of Ethics: expert guidance for professionals who treat addiction*, Geppert, C & Roberts, L, pp. 41-54, Hazelden, ISBN 9781592854929, Center City (MN).

Miller, P, Linteris, N & Forzisi, L. (2008). Is Groin Injecting an Ethical Boundary for Harm Reduction? *International Journal of Drug Policy*, Vol. 19, No. 6 (December 2008), pp. 486–91, ISSN 0955-3959.

Moore, D. (2007). Translating Justice and Therapy: the drug treatment court networks. *British Journal of Criminology*, Vol. 47, No. 1 (January 2007), pp. 42-60, ISSN 0007-0955.

Morgan, C, Kirkbride, J, Hutchinson, G, Craig, T, Morgan, K, Dazzan, P, Boydell, J, Doody, G, Jones, P, Murray, R, Leff, J & Fearon, P. (2008). Cumulative Social Disadvantage, Ethnicity and First-Episode Psychosis: a case-control study. *Psychological Medicine*,

Morgan, C, Burns, T, Fitzpatrick, R, Pinfold, V & Priebe, S. (2007). Social Exclusion and Mental Health: conceptual and methodological review. *British Journal of Psychiatry*, Vol. 191, No. 6 (December 2007), pp. 477-83, ISSN 0007-1250.

Morse, S. (2008). The Ethics of Forensic Practice: reclaiming the wasteland. *Journal of the American Academy of Psychiatry & the Law*, Vol. 36, No. 2 (June 2008), pp. 206-17, ISSN 1093-6793.

Muench, J & Hamer, A. (2010). Adverse Effects of Antipsychotic Medications. *American Family Physician*, Vol. 81, No. 5 (March 2010), pp. 617-22, ISSN 0002-838X.

National Coalition for the Homeless. (2009) *Mental Illness and Homelessness*, (July 2009), Retrieved from www.nationalhomeless.org/factsheets/Mental_Illness.pdf.

National Institutes of Health. (2010). *Summary of the FY 2011 President's Budget*. Retrieved from http://officeofbudget.od.nih.gov/pdfs/FY11/Summary%20of%20the%20FY%202011%20Presidents%20Budget.pdf.

Neale, J. (2008). Homelessness, Drug Use and Hepatitis C: a complex problem explored within the context of social exclusion. *International Journal of Drug Policy*, Vol. 19, No. 6 (December 2008), pp. 429-35, ISSN 0955-3959.

Nolan, J. (2003). Redefining Criminal Courts: problem solving and the meaning of justice. *American Criminal Law Review*, Vol. 40, No. 4 (Fall 2003), pp. 1541-65, ISSN 0164-0364.

Nussbaum, M. (1985). Finely Aware and Richly Responsible: moral attention and the moral task of literature. *Journal of Philosophy*, Vol. 82, No. 10 (October 1985), pp. 516-29, ISSN 0022-362X.

Onken, S, Craig, C, Ridgway, P, Ralph, R & Cook, J. (2007). An Analysis of the Definitions and Elements of Recovery: a review of the literature *Psychiatric Rehabilitation Journal*, Vol. 3, No. 1 (Summer 2007), pp. 9-22, ISSN 1095-158X.

Parker Jr., F & Burke, L. (2005). Employers, Ethics, and Managed Care. *Employee Benefit Plan Review*, Vol. 59, No. 9 (February 2005), pp. 7-11, ISSN 0013-6808.

Piko, B & Kovacs, E. (2010). Do Parents and School Matter? Protective factors for adolescent substance use. *Addictive Behaviors*, Vol. 35, No. 1 (January 2010), pp. 53-6, ISSN 0306-4603.

Pincus, H & McQueen, L. (2002). The Limits of an Evidence-Based Classification of Mental Disorders, In *Descriptions and Prescriptions: values, mental disorders, and the DSMs*, Sadler, J (ed.), pp. 9-24, Johns Hopkins University Press, ISBN 0801868408, Baltimore.

Pouncey, C & Lukens, J. (2010). Madness versus Badness: the ethical tension between the recovery movement and forensic psychiatry. *Theoretical Medicine & Bioethics*, Vol. 31, No. 1 (February 2010), pp. 93-105, ISSN 1386-7415.

Proulx, M, Leduc, N, Vandelac, L, Gregoire, J & Collin, J. (2007) Social Context, the Struggle with Uncertainty, and Subjective Risk as Meaning-Rich Constructs for Explaining HBP Noncompliance. *Patient Education & Counseling*, Vol. 68, No. 1 (September 2007), pp. 98-106, ISSN 0738-3991.

Radcliffe, P & Stevens, A. (2008). Are Drug Treatment Services Only for 'Thieving Junkie Scumbags'? Drug users and the management of stigmatized identities. *Social Science & Medicine*, Vol. 67, No. 7 (October 2008), pp. 1065-73, ISSN 0277-9536.

Radden, J & Sadler, J. (2010). *The Virtuous Psychiatrist*. Oxford University Press, ISBN 9780195389371, Oxford.

Rose, D, Thornicroft, G, Pinfold, V & Kassam, A. (2007). 250 Labels Used to Stigmatise People with Mental Illness. *BMC Health Services Research*, Vol. 7, No. 97 (June 2007), pp. 1-7, ISSN 1472-6963.

Ross, C & Goldner, E. (2009). Stigma, Negative Attitudes and Discrimination Towards Mental Illness within the Nursing Profession: a review of the literature. *Journal of Psychiatric & Mental Health Nursing*, Vol. 16, No. 6 (August 2009), pp. 558-67, ISSN 1351-0126.

Russell, B. (2008). An Integrative and Practical Approach to Ethics in Everyday Healthcare in *Risk Management in Canadian Health Care*, Dykeman, M & Dewhirst, K (eds.), pp. 9-13, Lexis-Nexis Canada, ISBN 978433443988, Toronto.

Rx&D. (2010). *Code of Ethical Practices*. Retrieved from

https://www.canadapharma.org/en/commitment/healthcare/pdfs/2010%20-%20Code%20of%20Ethical%20Practices_en.pdf.

Schmidt, N, Kotov, R & Joiner Jr., T. (2004). *Taxometrics: toward a new diagnostic scheme for psychopathology.* American Psychological Association, ISBN 1591471427, Washington DC.

Schulze, B. (2007). Stigma and Mental Health Professionals: a review of the evidence on an intricate relationship. *International Review of Psychiatry,* Vol. 19, No. 2 (January 2007), pp. 137-55, ISSN 0954-0261.

[Senate] Standing Committee on Social Affairs, Science and Technology. (2006). *Out of the Shadows at Last.* Retrieved from www.parl.gc.ca/39/1/parlbus/commbus/senate/com-e/soci-e/rep-e/pdf/rep02may06part1-e.pdf.

Shaffer, D, Hartman, J & Listwan, S. (2009). Drug Abusing Women in the Community: The impact of drug court involvement on recidivism. *Journal of Drug Issues,* Vol. 39, No. 4, (Fall 2009), pp. 803-28, ISSN 0022-0426.

Skorpen, A, Anderssen, N, Oeye, C & Bjelland, A. (2008). The Smoking Room as Psychiatric Patients' Sanctuary: a place for resistance. *Journal of Psychiatric and Mental Health Nursing,* Vol. 15, No. 9 (November 2008), pp. 728-36, ISSN 1365-2850.

Smith, T & Hirdes, J. (2009). Predicting Social Isolation Among Geriatric Psychiatry Patients. *International Psychogeriatrics,* Vol. 21, No. 1 (February 2009), pp. 50-9, ISSN 1041-6102.

Sokol, D. (2007). Ethicist on the Ward Round. *BMJ,* Vol. 335, No. 7621 (September 2007), pp. 670, ISSN 0959-8138.

Srebnik, D & Russo, J. (2008). Use of Psychiatric Advance Directives During Psychiatric Crisis Events. *Administration & Policy in Mental Health,* Vol. 35, No. 4 (July 2008), pp. 272-82, ISSN 0894-587X.

Srebnik, D, Rutherford, L, Peto, T, Russo, J, Zick, E, Jaffe, C & Holtzheimer, P. (2005). The Content and Clinical Utility of Psychiatric Advance Directives. *Psychiatric Services,* Vol. 56, No. 5 (May 2005), pp. 592-8, ISSN 1075-2730.

Stewart, D & DeMarco J. (2010) Rational Noncompliance with Prescribed Medical Treatment. *Kennedy Institute of Ethics Journal,* Vol. 20, No. 3 (September 2010), pp.

Stuhlmiller, C. (2005). Promoting Student Interest in Mental Health Nursing, *Journal of the American Psychiatric Nursing Association,* Vol. 11, No. 6 (December 2005), pp. 355-8, ISSN 1078-3903.

Sutherby, K, Szmukler, G, Halpern, A, Alexander, M, Thornicroft, G, Johnson, C & Wright, S. (1999). A Study of "Crisis Cards" in a Community Psychiatric Service. *Acta Psychiatrica Scandinavica,* Vol. 100, No. 1 (July 1999), pp. 56-61, ISSN 0001-690X.

Swanson, J, McCrary, S, Swartz, M, Elbogen, E & Van Dorn, R. (2006). Superseding Psychiatric Advance Directives: ethical and legal considerations. *Journal of the American Academy of Psychiatry & the Law,* Vol. 34, No. 3 (September 2006), pp. 385-94, ISSN 1093-6793.

Szasz, T. (2009). *Antipsychiatry: quackery squared.* Syracuse University Press, ISBN 9780815609438, Syracuse.

Szasz, T. (1976). *Schizophrenia: the sacred symbol of psychiatry.* BasicBooks, ISBN 9780465072224, New York.

Szasz, T. (1961). *The Myth of Mental Illness: foundations of a theory of personal conduct*. Harper & Row, ISBN 0060141964, New York.

Tessman, L. (2005). *Burdened Virtues: virtue ethics for liberatory struggles*. Oxford University Press, ISBN 9780195179156, Oxford.

Walker, D & Jackson J. (2011). The Effect of Legalized Gambling on State Government Revenue. *Contemporary Economic Policy*, Vol. 29, No. 1 (January 2011), pp. 101-14, ISSN 1465-7287.

Wilson, A & Beresford, P. (2002) Madness, Distress and Postmodernity, In *Embodying Disability Theory*, Corker, M & Shakespeare, T (eds.), pp. 143-58, Continuum, ISBN 0826450555, London (U.K.).

Wilson, H & Skodol, A. (1994). Special Report: DSM-IV: overview and examination of major changes. *Archives of Psychiatric Nursing*, Vol. 8, No. 6 (December 1994), pp. 340-7, ISSN 0883-9417.

Wilton, R. (2004). Putting Policy into Practice? Poverty and people with serious mental illness. *Social Science & Medicine*, Vol. 58, No. 1 (January 2004), pp. 25–39, ISSN 0277-9536.

Winkler, E. (2005). The Ethics of Policy Writing: how should hospitals deal with moral disagreement about controversial medical practices? *Journal of Medical Ethics*, Vol. 31, No. 10, (October 2005), pp. 559-66, ISSN 0306-6800.

World Health Organization. (2004). *The World Medicines Situation*. Retrieved from http://apps.who.int/medicinedocs/pdf/s6160e/s6160e.pdf.

World Health Organization. (2003). *Social Determinants of Health: the solid facts, second edition*. Wilkinson, R & Marmot, M. (eds.). Retrieved from www.euro.who.int/data/assets/pdf_file/0005/98438/e81384.pdf.

Zaner, R. (2004). *Ethics and the Clinical Encounter*. First Academic Renewal Press, ISBN 0788099396, Lima (OH).

4

Resource Allocation in Health Care

Giovanni Putoto and Renzo Pegoraro
Padova Teaching Hospital and Fondazione Lanza
Italy

1. Introduction

In many European countries where reforms of the welfare system are underway, reference is often made to the need to 'rationalise' the provision of health care. This term is generally used to refer to the need to organise healthcare effectively by reducing waste, containing costs, and ensuring that budgets are adhered to. Actions taken to achieve this are varied: some relate to the provision of services (for example, concentrating the provision of goods and services, redistributing health care workers); others require redefinition of the level of service provision (for example, avoiding hospital admission for conditions that can be treated in the clinic, or in day care); others rely on the application of the tools provided by *evidence based medicine* and *evidence based healthcare* to define the most effective medical care and interventions (for example, eliminating those procedures whose effectiveness is not supported by firm scientific evidence). All this is aimed at making healthcare provision more efficient and effective. Nevertheless, despite the efforts being made in this direction, it is becoming evident that rationalisation of healthcare provision is not sufficient in itself. The ageing population, the development of new and expensive technologies, the emergence of new diseases such as AIDS, Bovine Spongiform Encephalopathy (BSE), Severe Acute Respiratory Syndrome (SARS), and above all the rising expectations of healthcare users, are all leading to an unsustainable tension between demand and healthcare resources available.

Because it is not possible to provide everything to everyone, even by putting unacceptable pressure on present finances and by threatening provision for future generations, and since it is arguably socially unacceptable to leave the provision of healthcare to the free market, it is inevitable that certain choices be made. This implies a process of 'rationing', rather than 'rationalisation', that can be defined as 'the distribution of resources between programmes and persons in competition'. In the process of rationing, a series of crucial questions must be posed: What treatments or healthcare services should be provided to citizens? How should these services be distributed between members of a society amidst budgetary constraints? Who decides? How? On the basis of which criteria? The problem of rationing (also referred to as 'priority setting', or 'resource allocation') in healthcare is therefore a problem of the moral legitimacy of such choices; this chapter illustrates this. As challenges of rationing are not expected to change in the foreseeable future, at least not in principle, we will address future and present rationing challenges in health care similarly.

2. From implicit to explicit rationing

Traditionally, the many resource allocation decisions in healthcare were made in a non-explicit manner. Healthcare budgets were allocated to local authorities on a historical basis and doctors were given the task of deciding priorities for the provision of services. Today, increasingly, the choices made by politicians and professional healthcare managers must consider general and specific criteria in planning within budgetary constraints, and they are subject to scrutiny from a general public that is increasingly determined to see proper provision of healthcare in return for their taxes. But it is doctors that are seeing the greatest changes. The old pact that implicitly gave them the task of distributing healthcare resources according to their professional judgement is gone. In the medical world there is now an explicit requirement to account for the treatment choices made, and there are mechanisms for checking disparities in the provision of diagnostic and therapeutic services. These choices were once seen as strictly a matter of professional autonomy. A further change that is indicating a move to a more explicit form of rationing is the change in the once paternalistic doctor-patient relationship. A better educated population with easy access to healthcare information, that is increasingly aware of the need to become involved in decisions that concern their own body and health, and their associated rights to healthcare, is pushing to question doctors' decision making and to demand explanations of choices made to include or exclude certain conditions from healthcare provision. There are many cases of explicit rationing that are emerging in different European countries: one of the most widely discussed of these was the case of *Child B* in the United Kingdom, who was denied experimental therapy for leukaemia on the basis that it was prohibitively expensive and of unproven efficacy (Ham, 1999).

In general, there is some agreement that rationing should be more open and explicit, thus increasing accountability and the credibility of decision making. Despite this, a number of arguments have been posed against this, particularly that it may lead to instability in the health system and/or may cause harm to patients and the public. Others suggest that rationing is about decision making and should be considered a political process that is experimental and incremental.

3. Levels of rationing: macro, meso and micro

Healthcare rationing is a pervasive process that takes place at all levels and assumes various forms. Choices concern priorities, so that the rationing taking place at different levels of the public service through a hierarchy from high to low often constrains spending at the lower level. There are at least five levels at which choices are made:

- the level of funding to be allocated to health services
- the distribution of the budget between geographical area and services
- the allocation of resources to particular forms of treatment
- the choice of which patients should receive access to treatment
- decisions on how much to spend on individual patients

For convenience it is common to refer to three levels. The first ('macro') is the national or regional level, where the healthcare budget is decided. At this stage, decisions are made regarding increases in contributions, reductions in spending, or financing of particular programmes. Macro-decisions at a national level represent the key constraint within which

further divisions of funds between regions and local health providers are made according to formulae that vary from country to country.
The second ('meso') is the local level (regional or hospital), where resources are allocated to different functions and local authorities make decisions about local priorities. Such choices may involve the priorities attached to, for example, treatment services versus preventative medicine; particular patient groups, for example those with renal failure versus drug addicts; or certain hospital services, for example cancer services, versus other services such as respiratory care.
The third ('micro') level is the care level, where healthcare professionals make decisions about who, how, when, where and how to care for patients. This is a question of professional prerogative that can be limited by constraints from above, but never eliminated.

4. Decision makers and problems in reaching consensus: Who decides?

In societies where health services are funded and supplied principally via the state, cost increases and budgetary constraints impose difficult choices that influence the services that can be provided, the patients served and the circumstances of healthcare. The notion that public opinion can influence the decision making process has gained momentum. Taking note of public opinion obliges doctors, managers and politicians to take account of the concerns of the population, supports the formulation of objectives according to need, and favours social cohesion as well as civil identity. Many claim that without the agreement of the public, choices about rationing should never be effected, as they lack legitimacy. It is important to remember that public opinion about what services should be provided frequently differs from the opinions of doctors and healthcare managers. It is also important to note that in some jurisdictions, healthcare professionals other than doctors/physicians have a strong say in this matter.
Considering the tendency of healthcare providers to be sometimes unresponsive to the needs of society and inward looking, this develpoment of public involvment is to be considered a positive step. In a democratic society it is no longer acceptable to make decisions in the name of and on behalf of others without those others being informed and consulted. It is a matter of what we now call 'citizen rights'. Nevertheless, involving the public in decision making is a complex process, both in principle and in relation to the instruments that are used to gather public opinion. It is worth considering these limitations in order to mitigate their effects (Mossialos & King 1999):

- The public, in general, is not in possession of enough information to make decisions. Unless certain information is supplied regarding the effectiveness, risks, costs, and quality of life implications of interventions, along with the options for alternative treatments, decision makers cannot fully understand the problem
- There is a lack of familiarity with the debate on rationing, which would permit the public to be capable of assessing the questions presented
- The effect of bias in public opinion caused by emotional responses generated by a media that prefers sensationalist reporting to accurate presentaion of facts should not be underestimated, as shown by the Di Bella case in Italy (Benelli 2003).
- It is important to encourage the public to think in terms of public interest as a whole, for the common good over and above the good of individuals

- Even public representation, when it exists, can present its own problems. The inclusion or exclusion of certain groups or individuals can influence the range of attitudes and values expressed. One approach is to involve service users, another is to solicit general public opinion, or the opinion of institutional representatives. In the US state of Oregon, for example, groups of disabled persons rejected the first list of proposed funded treatments; they argued that the quality of life of disabled persons was undervalued by the Commission addressing their matter.
- It is also necessary to consider the level at which choices are made (Litvaa et al. 2002). At the system and program levels, informants generally tend to favour consultation, without taking responsibility for decisions, but with the guarantee that their contribution would be heard and that decisions taken following consultation would be explained. At the patient level, it may be that the public should participate only by setting criteria for deciding between potential beneficiaries of treatment, leaving the final say to the doctors and the patients involved (and other healthcare professionals and family involved).
- There are many methods that can be used to solicit public opinion. These include surveys, in-depth interviews, public meetings, community forums, focus groups and citizens' juries. This list is not exhaustive, but reflects a range of options available. Pros and cons in terms of time, costs, depth and breadth of analysis, discussion and deliberations should be taken into account.
- Regardless of the method used, the value of public participation in priority setting is largely dependent on the importance placed, by decision-makers, on the results of public consultation.

The participation of the public in setting priorities is key for legitimacy. It is an educational process that has to be encouraged and sustained. Public debate should be based on relevant information and accurate communication, be open and transparent with all stakeholders, and should make use of appropriate tools.

5. Methods of rationing

Methods of rationing that can be applied are many. In general they are classified as follows:
- *Selection*: Using this method, recipients of care are selected on the basis of clinical benefit they will obtain, or the amount of time required to treat them.
- *Denial*: This method involves the exclusion of certain patient populations because they are deemed unworthy, or because their needs are not seen as sufficiently important.
- *Deflection*: This involves referring patients to other institutions. It is a form of rationing when a patient's needs can be met by other health or social services.
- *Deterrence*: This involves deterring patients from accessing healthcare by the imposition of complex logistical/administrative requirements, such as inconvenient opening times, incomprehensible paperwork, and unhelpful staff. This type of rationing tends to disadvantage less educated and more vulnerable people.
- *Delay*: This method includes the use of waiting lists. It is the most recognised form of implicit rationing in healthcare, and discourages patients from accessing health services.
- *Dilution*: In this situation access to services is not denied, but the provision of services is reduced, such as the frequency of home visits.

- *Interruption*: This is the premature termination of a service or a treatment based on a maximum time limit for a given treatment, such as premature discharge from hospital or case closure.

Overall, these mechanisms of rationing are used by various decision makers, although only the first (selection) is formally endorsed. Often rationing is not deliberate or conscious, but is a means for professionals to cope with budgetary or other pressures. An alternative is the development of guidelines as a medium/long term solution.

6. Technical and distributive approaches to rationing

To make choices or establish priorities, certain criteria are required that reflect the most prevalent values in society. All countries that have embarked on this have stated the values on which they have based their choices. There are, in general, diverse principles that can guide a society's choices. These can be classified into technical criteria or distributive criteria. The first refer to the 'technical' qualities that services must possess in order to be included, such as efficiency, efficacy, and appropriateness. The others criteria are 'distributive' in nature, in that they help establish an order of priorities in the choice between different patient groups, such as relative benefit, and the rule of rescue.

7. Technical criteria

These are a prerequisite for any selection of priorities. For example, it is well established and accepted that healthcare interventions should be effective, efficient and appropriate. Such considerations can help in making choices, in as much as they help exclude those interventions that do not meet these criteria, but they are not enough in themselves to establish how many and which interventions to provide, and to whom.

- Effectiveness

The principle of effectiveness affirms that priority must be given only to those interventions that produce positive medical results. It is a principle that is intuitive and attractive in itself. The difficulties arise when one has to apply it and face up to the implications of this principle. According to some studies, the majority of surgical and medical procedures in use today are not based on scientific evidence of their effectiveness (85% according to the US Office of Technology Assessment). The scientific method for evaluating the effectiveness of healthcare treatments is based on the use of clinical research, and has as its gold standard the randomised controlled trial, the most rigorous assessment instrument, (hence real life circumstances) although it addressed efficacy rather than effectiveness. Despite the recent development of *evidence based medicine* and *evidence based health care* approaches and more refined instruments such as meta analysis, the criterion of effectiveness is not without its limitations. Above all, the collection and analysis of data about interventions is often expensive and may lead to ambiguous conclusions. Sometimes clinical research is not conducted with the required rigour, and frequently a treatment that may not be of general effectiveness may be appropriate in particular circumstances. To eliminate all procedures not demonstrated to be effective would therefore be unwise: even those treatments that are not scientifically well corroborated may sometimes be helpful.

- Efficiency

Efficiency is an economic concept. There are at least three types of efficiency that have been identified: technical, productive, and allocative.

Technical efficiency compares the resources required for a healthcare intervention (input) with the health benefits obtained (output). The relation must be as high as possible: maximum output compared with input, or minimal input compared with output. An example of technical efficiency is that of using 10mg of alendronate rather than 20mg of it in the treatment of osteoporosis since studies showed that the smaller dose achieved the same clinical results (assuming use of the smaller dose is less costly than use of the larger dose).

Productive efficiency is related to the possibility of choosing between two or more alternative treatments in relation to costs and results. Consider, for example, a policy of changing from maternal age screening to biochemical screening for Down's syndrome. The concept of productive efficiency refers to the maximisation of health outcome for a given cost, or the minimisation of cost for a given outcome. If the sum of the costs of the new biochemical screening program is smaller than or the same as the maternal age programme and outcomes are equal or better, then the biochemical program is productively efficient in relation to the maternal age program. In healthcare, productive efficiency enables assessment of the relative value for money of interventions with directly comparable outcomes.

Allocative efficiency refers to the destination of resources, which society makes available to various alternative uses, and defines as optimal the allocation that improves the health situation of an individual without compromising that of another.

The promise of the principle of efficiency, in its three forms, as a guide for defining choices, is attractive from an ethical point of view because it promises to deliver a greater volume of healthcare services at the same cost, and to make choices less painful. But problems emerge when applying this principle, in deciding the optimal allocation of scarce resources within a society. Economic theory in general has led to the development of various methods of evaluating the costs and benefits associated with different healthcare interventions, in particular analysis of cost/efficacy, cost/utility and cost/benefit. Criticisms of this approach lie not so much in the evaluation of costs, as in the notion of benefit and the consequences on health and above all, in distribution. In the cost/efficacy analysis, the results of a healthcare intervention are measured using indicators specific to the intervention or the disease treated (for example, reduction in infection rates, or rates of five year survival) and therefore do not allow a comparison between different illnesses, but only amongst alternative treatments for the same disorder (for example, medication compared to a surgical alternative). In cost/utility analysis this limitation has been overcome, to a certain extent, by the use of complex formulae such as QALYs (quality-adjusted life years) and DALYs (disability-adjusted life years), which tend to better reflect not only the cost of an intervention, but the quantity and quality of years of life productive/independent and functioning gained. This allows a comparison between different interventions for different illnesses and allows the creation of a 'league table' of interventions, based on these criteria. Evaluating cost/benefit can also include a monetary evaluation of the health gain, even an evaluation of the economic value of the extra years gained.

The limitations of these techniques are that from a technical point of view they are expensive, complex and difficult to carry out, and from an ethical point of view they mask serious value judgements beneath their seeming neutrality. The fact that scarce resources may be used to favour certain social groups to the exclusion of others solely on the basis of economic criteria causes much ethical and social concern.

- Appropriateness

According to traditional classifications of treatments, an appropriate treatment is one where the expected benefits exceed the expected negative effects (risks) associated with the treatment. One can distinguish between clinical and organisational appropriateness.

Clinical appropriateness – a treatment that is not effective cannot be appropriate, but a treatment that has been scientifically corroborated may still be inappropriate if carried out on a patient whose condition does not indicate its use in their particular circumstances. For some years the question of the appropriate use of interventions has been the subject of health service research, addressing the variation of the use of services. In the Unites States it is estimated that certain medical procedures (including coronary angiography, endoscopy, coronary artery by-pass surgery, and hysterectomy) have a rate of inappropriate use that ranges from 15-30%.

Organisational appropriateness refers to the type of service provision (inpatient ward, day unit, clinic) appropriate to the intervention offered in terms of patient safety and the most economic use of resources. With the introduction of such payment methods as diagnostic related groups (DRGs), the assessment of organisational appropriateness includes a review (known as a 'utilisation review') of clinical paperwork to evaluate the medical necessity of the treatment provided, the means of providing that treatment, and its duration. In this way the intervention and the appropriate timescale for such an intervention can be evaluated, and inappropriately long care identified.

8. Distributive criteria

Distributive criteria are a set of principles that establish an order of priority in the allocation of healthcare resources. They do not address the question of what must be guaranteed to individuals and society at large, but attempt to establish who (which individual, which social group) can have access to such resources.

- Need

In almost all methods of resource rationing there is an underlying principle of equality or justice, in which resources must be allocated according to need. A key element of justice requires that individuals with the same needs should receive the same treatment and that greater need takes priority over lesser need. The principle of equality requires that those with the greatest needs should have the greatest claim on resources. But how does one evaluate which need is greater than another? By whose evaluation: the doctor or the patient? Needs may be evaluated in terms of the consequences or results of interventions. A just society would have the moral obligation to provide for the needs of each citizen for treatment, but not for mere desires. Doctor and patient preferences may not coincide when, for example, decisions about quality versus quantity of life have to be made. Even if the concept of need is crucial, it remains ill defined and elastic. To what extent a society can satisfy needs is closely related to the resources available. Science can help in classifying needs on the basis of their consequences, independently of consideration of costs. The relation between needs and resources is, however, a political choice.

- Merit/demerit

According to the notion of merit, priority must go to those who deserve special consideration. For example, older people may deserve more attention as they have worked and paid their taxes for longer than anyone. Or children, because they have not yet had the chance to realise their human potential. Demerit is when judgments are made about lifestyle in relation to certain risk factors that may justify the restriction of the provision of health services. For example, heavy smokers, drug users and alcoholics may be deemed unworthy of receiving certain healthcare interventions unless they change their high-risk behaviour. The notion of merit/demerit is controversial if not unacceptable, as it contradicts the enlightenment tenet of the brotherhood (or more generally, siblinghood) of humanity.

- Risk

The concept of risk is similar to that of need and refers to the deterioration of a situation that could occur in the absence of an action or intervention. While the concept of need measures the deficit in well-being of an individual, that of risk evaluates the consequences of a non-intervention. The service providers possess the necessary information as to the relative grades of risk.

- Benefit

The communitarian sense of the principle of benefit is based on the discussion of collective good and the use of common resources. It is not the individual characteristics of need or risk that count have, but the final result for the community as a whole. Priority must be given to those who can gain the maximum benefit from an intervention (the 'capacity to benefit'). The underlying principle is that scarce resources must be used in such a way as to maximise the benefit not to the individual, but to the collective whole. According to this principle, it is immoral not to consider the costs associated with intervention, as this would mean ignoring sacrifices imposed on others.

- The rule of rescue

The duty to intervene when a life is in imminent danger cannot be avoided. According to this principle priority must be given to people in an emergency situation, or whose life is in danger. In healthcare, as in other sectors, the application of this principle is considered a fundamental indicator of our degree of civilisation. In fact, more importance is attached to the act of assisting than to the outcome of the intervention; this creates a practical difficulty, because it offers no assistance as to when to cease such interventions if the patient does not die. To apply the rule of rescue in all cases of need would lead to an unsustainably expensive system.

9. Theories of justice in healthcare

The technical criteria and particularly the distributive criteria that we have so far considered represent attempts to find some shared rational bases with which to deal with the problem of resource allocation in the health sphere. Apart from their apparent neutrality, they require a more or less explicit assumption of values. This in turn requires the consideration of theories of distributive justice, three in particular: *individual liberty, utilitarianism* and *egalitarianism*. These theories have profoundly different visions of the world, but are all inspired by two considerations that to a certain extent bind them together:

- Justice, while relevant to the individual conscience, is not restricted to the discretion of the individual, but represents the necessities of human coexistence
- Justice Relates to at least one of the following concepts: equality, liberty, responsibility, equity.

We will now examine different justice positions in more detail, both from a general point of view and in relation to the healthcare sphere.

The theory of individual liberty

This philosophical approach attaches the utmost importance to individual liberty rights. As a consequence, the state is required to support individual autonomy, both through rights that promote the notion and through promotion of a market economy. The market is left the task of redistributing resources in order to guarantee a level of dignified life for all, supporting individual expectations. The state becomes a discreet bystander in society where individual liberties take precedence, affording the fullest possible autonomy. For these reasons, in a 'pure' liberal state, there is no 'formal imperative' to support social solidarity. By definition the state is not obliged to tackle inequalities or to take on the task of supplying social services such as healthcare or education. In the healthcare sphere the results are as follows:

- There is no automatic 'right' to health for subjects
- The state is not morally obliged to provide any mechanism for the protection of health
- Health care is provided by means of a private contract between patient and healthcare provider; the patient pays for the service and the doctor/patient relationship reflects this
- The quality and amount of healthcare received is dependent on the ability of the patient to pay.

Utilitarian theory

The difficulties in the individual liberty theory lead to recourse to utilitarianism (or, more generally, consequentialism), where individual liberty rights are subordinated to the requirements to maximise *utility*, that is the state of 'maximum happiness and minimal misery', or 'the greatest happiness to the greatest number'. By definition, each action is judged on the basis of the amount of utility it generates: the objective is the best possible outcome for the largest amount of people for the minimum cost in terms of loss of utility. Utilitarianism thus inverts the relationship between individual and society, favouring the second. The state, in pursuing the goal of social utility, will favour the good of many over the individual.

The provision of a public healthcare system is in keeping with the theory as a whole, bearing in mind that the objective is the promotion of utility in terms of best possible health status for the maximum number of people. From a societal perspective, treating many patients who suffer from various conditions is viewed as equivalent to saving a few whose lives are in danger.

The theory of egalitarianism

The egalitarian model includes a multiplicity of positions, sometimes philosophically and politically far removed from each other. It brings together forms of socialism, social contract theory, and communitarianism. Egalitarianism attaches maximum importance to the equality of fundamental rights (to life, liberty, work, culture, and more) and to the conditions that support and protect these rights. Collective and societal needs take precedence over individual need in their theory, where upon public bodies have a pre-eminent role in their duty to protect and support the needy. This is the antithesis of individual libertarianism, as here a cooperative society is obliged to tackle inequality in all its forms:

'Social and economic inequality must satisfy two conditions: firstly, they must be attached to offices and positions open to all under conditions of fair equality of opportunity; secondly, such inequalities are justified only if they benefit the worst off' (Rawls 1999)
Egalitarian healthcare is based on the 'right to health' - protection and promotion of physical and mental integrity, healthcare and quality of life and of the environment are seen as positive rights. The state must take on the protection and promotion of these rights, through provision of universally accessible healthcare on the principle of solidarity.

10. The conflicts and limits of philosophical approaches

Theories of justice and their implications for the organisation of healthcare and the problems of rationing lend themselves to a series of considerations that illustrate both the strengths and weaknesses of such approaches.
Theories of *individual liberty* have the advantage of guaranteeing maximum individual freedom, but the price paid is high, particularly for those unable to participate fully in the marketplace and those whose individual autonomy is weakened (the poor, the elderly, the disabled, and others). Not only that, but the market imperative, far from promoting the well-being of many, rewards selfishness and highlights economic inequalities. Furthermore, freedom without responsibility is incomplete, the material and moral life ruled by laws of supply and demand, with the only aim being the attainment of individual freedom.
Utilitarianism has the advantage of subordinating individual advantages to the well being of the many, the key objective being to maximise collective utility. The theory is not without its criticisms, however. One of these is that in maximising utility to the collective whole, there is potential to ignore the needs of the individual. There are also difficulties in defining utility, given that this is a subjective term (as wanted in quality of life assessments). The values involved, the burdens of expensive treatment and the clinical benefit derived for the patient are incommensurable (not capable of being compared with each other) unless there is a similar treatment alternative to use as comparator. Where there is no alternative, the application of a utilitarian evaluation often creates more problems than it resolves.
Egalitarianism seeks maximum social justice and protection of rights, but this theory also incurs criticisms. First, what is the foundation of this equality? Based on the social mechanism we want to refer to, social rights may be embedded in a more or less solid foundation. In the case of the social contract, rights are normally attributed to members of society or, by the same vein, are drawn from them. Yet social rights could also be attributed, regardless of a social agreement, as fundamental human entitlements that cannot be questioned, for example by the majority rule. Secondly, there is a risk that social dynamics could prevail over the individual, forcing the latter to accept priorities and objectives that are opposed to his or her own rights.
To conclude this part, when referring to rationing in health care, it can be argued that in pluralistic societies there are continuous tensions and confrontations about what distributive justice is about and how it can be guaranteed to citizens. An agreement based on the philosophical approaches outlined above is likely to be unachievable, thus it is necessary to explore other solutions to the problem of rationing of health care resources.

11. The ethico-procedural approach

Normative approaches are important as they help identify fundamental values that are at the core of political decision making, but they are not enough in themselves, as we saw that different theories lead to different conclusions and there is no consensus on which is the correct approach to take. Added to that is the fact that they are too abstract to be applied as such to the reality of the world of healthcare institutions. Empirical approaches are sometimes helpful, because they help identify what has been done and what could be done, but not what should be done. In the absence of a broad consensus on the acceptability of various guiding principles for the allocation of resources, the problem of 'fair' distribution becomes a question of 'procedural justice'. An ethico-procedural approach requires a decision making process that allows agreement on what is legitimate and fair in terms of rationing. Rather than concentrating on principles and values that should underpin decision making, the ethico-procedural approach asks how such decisions are made. It involves a shifting of perspective from content to process. The rationale on which the ethico-procedural approach is based is as follows: irrespective of the financing or provision of health services, legitimate authority is conferred by the influence of the democratic process on the system. A well known ethico-procedural approach is *'accountability for reasonableness'* (Daniel & Sabin 2002). The conditions essential to the application of this approach are as follows:

1. *Publicity condition*: decisions regarding both direct and indirect limits to care and their rationales must be publicly accessible.
2. *Relevance condition*: the rationales must rest on evidence, reasons, and principles that all fair minded parties (managers, clinicians, patients, and consumers in general) can agree are relevant to deciding how to meet the diverse needs of a covered population under necessary resource constraints.
3. *Appeals condition*: there is a mechanism for challenge and dispute resolution regarding limit setting decisions, including the opportunity for revising decisions in light of further evidence or arguments.
4. *Enforcement condition*: there is either voluntary or public regulation of the process to ensure that the first three conditions are met.

The advantages of this approach are many. For instance, there is an educational aspect. All parties to the decision can appreciate the value of debate and deliberation in achieving a fair decision under resource constraints. Furthermore, *'accountability for reasonableness'* occupies a middle ground between implicit rationing and explicit rationing. In a similar fashion to the implicit approach, the principles on which the decision is made do not have to be disclosed in advance; in contrast, as in the explicit approach, there is an appeal to greater transparency in disclosing the reasons for decisions on rationing resources.

12. International experiences

At the international level, there are three basic strategies for rationing that have emerged. The first (and until now the only example of its kind) is that employed by Oregon (USA), which tackled two issues together: which treatments, and how much treatment, should the state provide to its citizens whilst acting within its budgetary restraints? It is the most explicit and radical form of rationing to date. A second strategy is that of the Netherlands and Sweden, which defined a set of principles on which to base a healthcare package of available treatments for eligible citizens (the Netherlands), or to define priorities in the supply of healthcare (Sweden). Neither country has managed to produce a list of available treatments. A third strategy is that adopted by New Zealand and Great Britain, who are not so much concerned with general principles as with putting into place a continual process of drawing up guidelines and advice on appropriate treatment, supporting their view that rationing should take place at the local and individual (micro) level.

Oregon

The US state of Oregon was the first to explicitly and fundamentally address problems of rationing in healthcare. Following the death from leukaemia of a child who was denied a transplant, the authorities set up a commission in 1989, the Health Services Commission, to make recommendations on how the government funded Medicaid program could be extended to include a section of the population who were not covered, and how to set priorities within the Medicaid program itself. Having unsuccessfully tried an exclusively technical approach (cost effectiveness analysis), they turned to a method that paired disease with treatments and ordered these according to the gravity of the disease. Adjustments were made to the list, according to what the Commission viewed as 'reasonable' and taking into account the results of a public consultation. The 'Oregon Plan' was put into practice in 1994, financing 565 treatments of the 696 listed. This list has since been amended and changes were made to the originally identified priorities. The abandonment of the technical approach, debated furiously by the medical profession and the public alike, has become a symbol and a learning opportunity for many countries faced with difficult choices in rationing.

The Netherlands

The Dutch government set up a Government Committee on Choices in Healthcare in 1990, with the mandate remit of examining the problem of choices in healthcare and identifying criteria for drawing up a basic package of healthcare treatments that should be offered to all citizens with the necessary state or private health insurance. In their report, delivered in 1991, the Committee adopted a broad approach, with a method for evaluating the necessity and availability of treatments, using four criteria/filters:

- Necessity
- Efficacy
- Efficiency
- Individual responsibility

The report also dealt with issues such as technological developments, waiting lists, the appropriateness of treatment, and public involvement in priority setting. The Committee, however, did not chose to produce a list of treatments for inclusion in the basic package, but limited itself to applying the principles to a few controversial cases (in-vitro fertilisation, homeopathic medicine, dental care for adults, sports injury services, care of the elderly).

Sweden

The Swedish Parliamentary Priorities Commission was set up in 1992 to 'discuss the role of health services in its social context and to outline the fundamental ethical principles that should guide the necessary prioritisation of resources'. An interim report entitled 'No Easy Choices' was published in 1993 and circulated for comment. The Commission identified two types of approache to the problem of priority setting: a clinical approach based on patient need, and a politico-administrative approach where scarce resources needed to be considered. An interesting feature of the Swedish deliberations was the development of an ethical platform based on certain principles to guide choices about priorities:

- The human dignity principle
- The principle of need and solidarity
- The cost/efficiency principle

The final report did not contain a detailed list of services to be included or excluded, but it did group treatments into five classes of descending priority. This approach is a method for assisting in establishing priorities and helping those responsible to make decisions.

New Zealand

In 1992 a National Advisory Committee on Core Health Services was set up in New Zealand to 'make explicit which services everyone should have access to, in acceptable terms and without unreasonable waiting times'. The practical difficulties in drawing up a definitive list led the Committee to identify as essential those services already provided, because these were deemed to be so as the 'result of many years of reasonable good sense, decisions founded on principle'. The Committee to developed guidelines for services of general application, those with high costs, or those that are delivered in high volume. The guidelines are shared at conferences, and efforts to involve the public in the debate are notable.

Great Britain

In Great Britain there has been no national committee set up to address the problem of priority setting in healthcare. The task is delegated at a local level, and local authorities must determine an annual plan of services they wish to provide. Some have been more explicit in recent years about which services they will provide, albeit thus far restricting access to marginal treatments such as tattoo removal. At a national level there is an agency that evaluates treatments and develops guidelines - the National Institute for Health and Clinical Excellence - and another that looks at service performance - the Health Care Commission.

Developing countries

Developing countries who have limited resources more than developed countries, are obliged to make difficult choices in terms of healthcare provision and who to provide it to. A specific example is the provision of antiretroviral treatment for AIDS sufferers in Africa. Scarce resources, even when accounting for international help, do not permit universal access to these drugs: choices have to be made. Governments can make such choices on the basis of financial, socio-economic or medical criteria. As an alternative, or in conjunction, they may be allocated on the basis of less formal, unfair criteria such as individual preferences of decision makers, or political considerations (Rosen 2005). Developing countries are advised by the World Bank to direct resources to public health programs on the basis of economic and cost efficiency considerations, using tools such as the *Disability Adjusted Life Years* tool (World Bank 1993). In any case, the same considerations need to be taken into account: who decides? On the basis of which criteria? On what values are decisions based? How democratic is the decision making process?

12. Conclusion

International experiences serve to highlight yet again just how difficult the issue of rationing in healthcare is. Every country we have considered has found its own way to set priorities. There is no consensus on principles, or on the methodologies used to make choices. General principles, when they have to be applied in a practical way at a local or individual level, have to be interpreted in light of circumstances and there is an ever-present ambiguity in this application. It is not possible to predict all the situations in which the rules will have to be applied, so a certain level of discretion and interpretation is required. All this confirms that there are no easy solutions at hand (Holm 1998).

Coulter and Ham (2001) summarized international experience with health care priority setting, and concluded:

'there is a need to strengthen institutional processes in which decisions are taken; priority setting processes must be transparent and accountable; clinical guidelines are increasingly being used as a priority setting tool, but fair processes are needed for guidelines, just as for priority setting more generally; the politics of rationing favours muddling through and the evasion of responsibility, but this is unsustainable in an era of increasing public awareness about policy making; priority setting policy making is an exercise in policy learning; and "accountability for reasonableness" is a leading ethical framework for priority setting in institutions'.

Accordingly, a strategy for improving priority setting in health care entails improving priority setting processes using guidance such as that provided by the "accountability for reasonableness" approach. Without analysis and debate about public policy, people and institutions can make arbitrary decisions about access to treatment, and implicit rationing can foster both inequity and inefficiency.

13. References

Benelli E. (2003). The role of the media in steering public opinion on healthcare issues. *Health Policy,* Vol. 63, No. 2, (February, 2003), pp.179-186, ISSN 0168 8510.

Coast, J., Donovan, J., Litva, A., Eyles, J., Morgand, K., Shepherd, M. & Tacchie, J. (2002). 'If there were a war tomorrow, we'd find the money': contrasting perspectives on *the rationing of health care. Social Science & Medicine , Vol.54, No.12, (June 2002), pp.1839–1851, ISSN 0277 9536.*

Coulter A. & Ham C. (eds.) (2001). *The Global Challenge of Health Care Rationing.* Philadelphia: Open University Press, Buckingham. ISBN 0 335 20463 5.

Daniels N. & Sabin E. (2002) *Setting Limits Fairly.* New York: Oxford University Press. eISBN 019514936X, ISBN 9780195149364, New York USA.

Gibson L., Martin D. & Singer P. (2005). Priority setting in hospitals: fairness, inclusiveness, and the problem of institutional power differences. *Social Science & Medicine,* Vol. 61, No. 11, (December, 2005), pp. 2355-2362, ISSN 0277-9536.

Ham C. (1999). Tragic choices in health care: lessons from the *Child B* case. *BMJ,* Vol.319, No. 7219, (June, 1999), pp.1258-1261, ISSN 0959 8138.

Holm S. (1998). Goodbye to the simple solutions: the second phase of priority setting in health care. *BMJ,* Vol. 317, No. 7164, (October, 1998),pp. 1000-1002, ISSN 0959 8138.

Klein R. (1993). Dimensions of rationing: Who should do what?. *BMJ*, Vol.307, No. 6899, (July, 1993), pp.309-311, ISSN 0959 8138.

Klein R. (1995). Priorities and rationing: Pragmatism or principles?. *BMJ*, Vol. 311, No. 7008, (September, 1995), pp. 761-762, ISSN 0959 8138 .

Klein R., Day, P. & Redmayne, S. (1996). *Managing scarcity*. In Ham .C (ed.) State of Health Series. Buckingham: Open University Press.

Litva A., Coast, J., Donovan, J., Eyles J., Shepherd, M., Tacchif J., Abelsong J, Morgane K. (2002). 'The public is too subjective': public involvement at different levels of health-care decision making. *Social Science & Medicine*, Vol. 54, no.12, (June, 2002), pp.1825–1837, ISSN 0277 9536

Mossialos E. & King D. (1999). Citizens and rationing: analysis of a European survey. *Health Policy*, Vol. 49, No.1-2, (October, 1999), pp. 75–135, ISSN 0168 8510.

Rawls J. (1971) *A Theory of Justice*. Cambridge: Harvard University Press, ISBN 0 674 01772 2.

Rosen, S., Sanne, I., Collier, A. &Simon, J.L. (2005). Hard choices: rationing antiretroviral therapy for HIV/AIDS in Africa". *Lancet*, Vol.365, No. 9456, (January, 2005), pp. 354-356, eISSN 1474 547X

Spagnolo A. et al (2004) *Etica e giustizia in sanità*. Milano: Mc Graw Hill 2004. World Bank (1993) World Development Report: Investing in Health. New York: Oxford University Press.

Deber R., Wiktorowicz M., Leatt P., Champagne F. (1994). Technology acquisition in Canadian hospitals: how is it done, and where is the information coming from?" *Healthcare Management Forum*, Vol. 7, No.4, pp. 18–27, ISSN 0840 4704 .

Deber R., Wiktorowicz M., Leatt P., Champagne F. (1995). Technology acquisition in Canadian hospitals: how are we doing? *Healthcare Management Forum*, Vol.8, No. 2, pp. 23–28, ISSN 0840 4704 .

Martin D.K., Shulman K., Santiago-Sorrell P., Singer P.A. (2003). Priority setting and hospital strategic planning: a qualitative case study. *Journal of Health Services Research and Policy*, Vol. 8 No.4, (2003), pp. 197–201 ISSN 1355-8196, .

Madden S., Martin D.K., Downey S., Singer P.A. (2005). Hospital priority setting with an appeals process: a qualitative case study and evaluation. *Health Policy*, Vol. 73, No. 1, (July, 2005), pp.10–20, ISSN 0168 8510.

Hope T., Hicks N., Reynolds D.J.M., Crisp R., Griffiths S. (1998). Rationing and the Health Authority. *BMJ*, Vol. 317, No.7165, (October, 1998), pp. 1067–9, ISSN 0959 8138.

Mitton C. & Donaldson C. (2002). Setting priorities in Canadian Regional Health Authorities: a survey of key decision makers. *Health Policy*, Vol. 60, No. 1, (April, 2002), pp. 39–58, ISSN 0168 8510.

Singer P.A., Martin D.K., Giacomini M., Purdy L. (2000). Priority setting for new technologies in medicine: a qualitative case study. *BMJ* , Vol.321, No.7272, (November, 2000), pp. 1316–8, ISSN 0959 8138

Foy R., So J., Rous E., Scarffe J.H. (1999). Perspectives of commissioners and cancer specialists in prioritising new cancer drugs: impact of the evidence threshold. *BMJ*, Vol. 318, No. 7181, (February, 1999), pp. 456–9, ISSN 0959 8138.

Martin D.K., Pater J.L., Singer P.A. (2001) "Priority setting decisions for new cancer drugs: a *qualitative study". Lancet, Vol. 358, No. 9294, (November, 2001), pp. 1676–81,* ISSN 0140 6736.

5

Ethics and Medically Assisted Procreation: Reconsidering the Procreative Relationship

Laurent Ravez
Associate Professor at the University of Namur,
Director of the Interdisciplinary Center on Law, Ethics and Health Sciences
Belgium

1. Introduction

Since the birth of Louise Brown, the first 'test-tube baby' in the history of humanity, in July 1978, criticisms of MAP have not ceased. These criticisms are generally of two types. The first relates to the medico-technical dimension of MAP and questions the effectiveness and the safety of these biotechnologies. The second, which I will discuss here, relates to the ethical dimension of MAP.

I will initially review the ethical criticisms of MAP, particularly in the Francophone literature (although this is not significantly different in the Anglophone literature), and suggest a way of classifying them, before going on to show the limits of such a classification. These criticisms can be grouped into three categories: the medicalization of procreation, the upheaval in the structures of filiation, and the status of the embryo. We will see that, although this criticism is enlightening in certain cases, it is often excessive and, at the same time, overlooks the effectiveness of procreation technologies in relieving the suffering of sterile couples, as argued in previous work of mine (Ravez, 2006).

The suffering of the patients is an essential element in the ethical evaluation of MAP, but it is not sufficient to construct a satisfactory axiological framework. I will show that such a framework is essential. I will propose three components of such a framework, taking into account the limits of criticism addressed at MAP, but also the limits of MAP itself.

2. The "medicalization" of procreation

The "medicalization" of procreation, of which some accuse MAP, is demonstrated through two professional attitudes:

1. Formulation of the desire for a child as a need to be satisfied immediately,
2. Construal of sterility as pathology.

By "formulation of the desire for a child…", I mean a deep misunderstanding of the complexity which drives two human beings to join together and from which sometimes a child emerges as a symbol of this union. For those who denounce this misunderstanding, it is particularly limiting to imagine that the human desire for a child is only or mostly biological, while trying to resolve possible mechanical failures that may have lead to this sterility. To illustrate this, I quote Genevieve Delaisi de Parseval who wrote: "It is in the mind that children are conceived"(Delaise de Parseval & Verdier, 1985, p.20).

Viewed as a need, the child, when it is desired, must be obtained as fast as possible and under the best possible conditions. *Desire* is formulated as a *need* everyone has the *right* to have fulfilled. In this view, sterility constitutes an obstacle to the need to have a child, which reproductive medicine has the duty to alleviate. Many authors that are critical of MAP argue that "pathologizing" sterility is likely to eliminate the psychological suffering which is sometimes the origin of this desire. It may be better to listen initially to what couples with procreative difficulties are trying to say, before launching into a series of biomedical procedures. In other words, sterility should be considered as a call to listen to the relationship rather than or only as a call to medical techniques and procedures.

3. Upheaval in the social structures of filiation

MAP is also regularly accused in the Francophone literature of upsetting the traditional structures of filiation, thus threatening to destroy the foundation of the human family.

Artificial insemination by sperm donor (AID) makes it possible to dissociate biological procreation and social filiation (Mehl, 1999). With this dissociation, the social father is no longer necessarily the biological father of the children carried by his partner. Socially speaking, this situation is not new. Adoption or adultery may also produce such situations. But the novelty is found in the involvement of science, specifically biotechnologies, in this dissociation.

The development of in vitro fertilization (IVF) with donor gametes (ovules and/or spermatozoa) has reinforced the difference between these two modes; biological procreation and social filiation. It has been suggested that you can make a child today by rallying different people to the cause and without anyone of them having sexual relations with anyone else (Malherbe, 1997). You only need the collaboration of: one *genetic father*, who provides the spermatozoa, one *genetic mother* for the ovules, one *surrogate mother* providing her uterus, one *adoptive mother* who will become the socially recognized mother of the child, one *surrogate father*, companion of the surrogate mother, and one *adoptive father* who will become the legal father.

Given such dissociation of the elements of procreation, there is fear that the very basis of our life as a society will be undermined. We have an amalgam of ideas concerning paternity, situated somewhere between *bloodlines*, i.e., the parent of a child is the source of the biological conception, and the *will*–, i.e., the parent of a child is the source of the desire for, and the choice of, a child. Behind these problems, we find a question present in social anthropology: does one become a father through conception or filiation? In all human societies, as regards filiation, there may be a primacy of the social over the biological. The anthropologist Francoise Héritier states: "To sum up, there has never been a human society up to the present that is based solely on the biological sense of filiation, or that would give a purely biological relationship the same weight as the social sense of filiation" (Héritier, 1996, p.258) . Actually, one could advance the idea that, in the view of social anthropology, not only has the cleavage between *social filiation* and *biological filiation* existed everywhere and always, but that this cleavage makes it possible to mitigate a situation of sterility, which is often badly accepted socially.

4. The status of the embryo

As for the status of the embryo, there are many controversies about it. Opinion n°18 (September 16, 2002) of the Consultative Committee of Bioethics of Belgium (CCB)

regarding research on human embryos *in vitro* notes the difficulty of agreeing on the moral status of the embryo. It highlights five possibilities.
The first possibility is "intentionalist" or "externalist" and is defended by those who state that the moral status of the embryo depends on the intentions of its (biological) parents. According to this approach, the human embryo cannot be regarded as a person in its own right unless it is part of a project of parenthood. Such a project is absent in the case of supernumerary embryos or embryos created for experimental purposes. The second possibility is to respect the embryo as a person as soon as the ovule has been fertilized; this position is described as "internalist" or "creationist". A third possibility offers moral status to the embryo starting on the 15th day of development. The fourth possibility corresponds to the oppinions defended in 1984 and 1986 by the National Consultative Ethics Committee for Health and Life Sciences (CCNE) in France, according to which the embryo is a potential person, i.e., it is not an actual person, but it has the potential to become one and must be respected for this potentiality. The last possibility is known as "gradualist", in the sense that the human embryo has variable moral status according to its degree of development: a 39 week foetus will have to be respected and protected more than a 10 weeks old embryo.
The question of the moral status of the embryo is of paramount importance, because the MAP techniques require the sacrifice of many embryos to carry out experiments. If we regard the embryo as a person from the very first stages of its development, it is clear that these experiments should cease.
Mehl writes: "In the end, scientists characterize the humanity of an embryo, not on an essential definition, but rather by what they want to do with it. Paradox: in the past, science tested the embryo to know what it could do with it. And now, it gives the embryo a status in function of what it wants to do with it - authorize abortion, do research… So, the status of the embryo by scientists seems fundamentally opportunistic" (Mehl, 1999, p.90-1). This accusation of "opportunism" seems to structure the paper: "The Random Embryo" [L'embryon aléatoire] (Hermitte, 1990). Her criticisms remind us of the moral principle: the end does not justify the means. Applied to our subject, this principle could mean: whatever 'benefits' MAP may bring to couples, it is at the unjustifiable expense of some embryos. On the other hand, those embryos may not exist from the start without MAP.

5. Suffering denied

Such criticisms help us recognize the weaknesses or even the dangers involved in the new MAP techniques. Nevertheless, whatever the relative merits of such criticisms, they lack insight into the suffering of sterile couples and into the effectiveness of new MAP techniques to relieve this suffering.
Many clinicians note the suffering of sterile couples that want a child. The symptoms of this distress are reminiscent of those of clinical depression. Muriel Flis-Trèves, a psychiatrist who worked in the team of Prof Frydman ('father' of the first French 'test-tube baby'), writes on this subject: "The suffering which accompanies the diagnosis [of sterility] is intense. It is often followed by a sudden withdrawal from the interests of daily existence, including work, leisure, and even temporarily from sexual activities". For men, Luc Roegiers notes that the principal elements of this depression relate to "self doubt, his sexual prowess, his capacity to transmit his genome" (Roegiers, 1994, p.169).

Confronted with this suffering, MAP can bring relief to the suffering couple, quite simply by providing the long awaited child. Positive testimony from couples helped by MAP is much more difficult to find than complaints when the treatment fails. After the pregnancy has finally started, couples often forget the particular circumstances which ushered in their dearest wish. Muriel Flis-Trèves writes: "As soon as she becomes pregnant, the woman who had recourse to MAP aspires to become a mother like any other. Her pregnancy is now 'banal' and she is confronted with the same anxieties, joys and hopes as all other women" (Flis- Trèves, 1998, p.191). Béatrice Koeppel, a psychologist specializing in sterility has the same position: "The first or second year after the birth of Amandine, the pregnancies with IVF [in-vitro fertilization] seemed still extraordinary. This is not at all any longer the case. On the contrary, the pregnancy is seen as banal. And it is what people appreciate with MAP: to be like any future mother, to complain about restrictions, to consult books avidly, to be no different from their peers" (Koeppel, 2000, p. 167-168). Soon after the pregnancy is underway, even the idea of sterility becomes unbearable to many couples helped by MAP, which makes discussion of their (former) sterility very difficult.

6. A "blank cheque" for MAP?

If the suffering of the sterile couples constitutes an essential element of the case for MAP, it is still not reasonable to give the medical staff a "blank cheque". It is important not to lose sight of the fact that this kind of treatment is extremely dependant on technical and scientific advances, in particular on biotechnologies. As Jacques Ellul – French sociologist who had a great influence on the Francophone philosophy of technology - states, techno scientific development is mainly guided by what we could call "technical imperatives" or "the technician's imperative", which can be summarized as: "Anything that is possible technically, should be done" (Ellul, 1954, pg, 122). The technology in itself is not unethical, but is in fact outside of ethics, that is to say ethically undetermined as to the question of its development.

Without ethical limits, MAP runs the risk of exacerbating the very problem it is trying to resolve: the suffering of sterile couples. We have to acknowledge the successes of MAP; we must also consider its failures and the suffering it may cause. This is suffering that the authors who criticize MAP denounce, that is to say the suffering of couples for whom MAP failed to offer the baby desired and for whom distress was increased further with the procedure. On this point, G. Delaisi de Parseval writes: "[...] medical procedures regarding infertility [...] almost always produce sexual dysfunctions: taking of temperatures, scheduled or forbidden sexual intercourse, analysis, exams, invasive treatments that interfere with sexual desire or the achievement of intercourse, anxiety induced by medicalization, [...] sometimes compromise the balanced relationship within the couple" (Delaisi de Parseval, 1985, p. 61).

On the one hand, we must recognize the effectiveness of MAP in fighting the plague of sterility. On the other, we must avoid an approach which would justify the use of any and all bio-technologies as regards human procreation, under the pretext of possible therapeutic benefits. It is clear, however, that such an effort at clarity can only be effective given an ethical framework, which is acceptable for both experts and patients, as well as for policy makers. Today, MAP is integrated in the medical scene and I don't intend to call into question its provision, as do numerous authors. But, while accepting the principle of MAP, it is important to optimize its provision, not only on a technical level but also on an ethical level.

7. Rethinking the procreation relationship and outlining a new axiological framework

It would seem worthwhile to look further at the following framework:

1. Listen to those suffering from sterility, without necessarily endorsing everything they say;
2. Respect the complexity of the gift of life;
3. Consider technical and scientific advances not as an end in themselves, but as a means to serve the couple's desire for a child (keeping resource constraints in mind).

8. Listening to those suffering from sterility, without necessarily endorsing everything they say

The challenge here is to encourage the parties involved in the area of reproductive medicine to take the suffering and the stress related to sterility seriously, while leaving open the question of whether or not this suffering is the cause or the consequences of this sterility. We find an illustration of this position in the words of M. Bydlowski, one of the experts on the psychology of infertility in France: "Years of work of consultation on infertility have confronted us with the suffering of patients. [...] Their distress is the consequence of their infertility. However, it appeared to us that this suffering often exists before the symptomatic demand: the infertility would then be the testimony of that suffering" (Bydlowski, 2000a, p. 119). If the infertility is the result of mental distress, any benefit which MAP might cause may not eliminate the existential malaise; this would need to be heard and explored before or unrelated to launching a parenting project. Experts should find and use the means to differentiate among the requests for a child which they receive, to identify what are calls for help from women or couples for whom MAP is a band-aid for a wounded existence. Imagine a request for help, directed to a doctor, to have a child, from a patient who in fact desperately seeks psychological healing, a healing that may not occur even when a child might finally be born.

To illustrate this point, I turn to E. Jéronymidès, a therapist accompanying women with procreative difficulties. She relates the case of a consultation with a woman looking for medical assistance for secondary sterility. After two sessions, the patient, who had a very difficult relationship with her husband, disappeared from care for several years. The therapist later met her by chance. "Four years later, I bumped into her. She remembered me and seemed happy to speak to me. She told me that she now had a two month old little boy. She had him naturally, without MAP. She did not plan it, did not program it in any way. Then she recalled that she had not contacted the hospital or MAP programme at the time, because her father had fallen seriously ill. He had ended up being hospitalised and he died of cancer. 'That's the reason', she told me, 'that I didn't return to see you any more. I had a lot of difficulty accepting the death', she told me in a very serious tone, 'I haven't gotten over it yet and I'm not sure I ever will. It's very difficult losing your father. I was really very attached to him'. She said that she doesn't breast feed her child because she has a lot of work and that she has to leave her house everyday. The tone she uses about the birth of the baby is neutral, with a hint of bitterness. It's as though the arrival of the child, and his presence with her could not, despite everything, fill the place of the loss of her father" (Jéronymidès, 2001, p. 54).

In other words, the suffering expressed at the fertility clinic can mask existential difficulties - discord within the couple, difficulties with their parents, an unhappy childhood (Bydlowski, 2000, Ravez, 2006) – that MAP, as such, has no way of detecting or resolving, simply because MAP is a technology designed to treat biological dysfunctions. In that context, the risk is high that professionals will assist the couple with techniques they actually don't want. An interdisciplinary approach at the MAP clinic, using a team of doctors, nurses, psychologists, social workers and others can reduce this risk.

9. Respecting the complexity of the gift of life

To give life, whether it comes "naturally" or with the assistance of medical science, does not only involve an efficient mobilization of gametes, a physiological process or a properly functioning organism. The family context, the psychological aspects and the genealogy are essential and must not be set aside. These elements are determining factors for a healthy parental relationship. Bydlowski wrote: "The human child will result from the unique mixture of the biological programming specific to the species - nucleic acids, molecules, cells - with the pre-existent parental psyche – the secret desires, dreams, memories, and words" (Bydlowsi, 2000b, p.24). Life presents a genetic or a biological dimension, but is also given to the child in the midst of lived complexity, emotional and generational relations created by their parents. MAP often undermines this complexity, as Brigitte-Fanny Cohen, a famous French journalist who engaged herself in a MAP procedure, states: "My feeling, at least, is that for [...] agents of MAP, gynaecologists and biologists, I was just a womb and ovaries, at best, a rate of FSH, a number of follicles or oocytes" (Cohen, 2001, p.67).

In the same manner, MAP can sometimes ignore important stakeholders such as husbands or other partners and grandparents, due to the desire for a child. Husbands may not be considered as agents in their own right in the procreative project, and are sometimes treated as simple carriers of gametes. As the gynaecologist Pierre Fonty wrote provocatively: "These men have the impression of being reduced to the rank of a sperm machine that produces on demand, and to no longer being seen as beings animated by the desire for their partner, having their own desires and sexual instincts" (Fonty, 2003, p. 100).

However, the situation is gradually changing, as certain practitioners of MAP seem to be more aware lately of the non-biological importance of the father considerations are now more often invoked. Delaisi de Parseval speaks about the "father who became a father because of his own father's regard of him; in short a father who lives through the experience of paternity that is paradoxically, not very different from that of maternity" (Delaisi de Parseval, 2003, p.110). Thus clearly "to be a father implies referring to their own role as a son" (Clerget, 2003, p. 121). Paternity and fatherhood include both inheritance and transmission.

10. Considering technical and scientific advances not as an end in themselves, but as a means to serve the couple's desire for a child (keeping resource constraints in mind)

Contrary to some critiques of MAP, MAP offers increasingly effective ways for sterile couples to have the desired child. But public health education is needed in relation to

MAP. The methods and techniques of MAP need to be seen as ways of helping couples have children and not as the cure for distress and angst in modern life. MAP does not offer happiness, but does create the technical conditions to allow the couple's happiness to be expressed through and with the birth of a child. In other words, we can't expect MAP to offer love, a sense of balance, or harmony within the couple. Quite the contrary, if the couple is fragile, the difficulties of MAP are likely to worsen the situation further. To address this, an on-going dialogue should occur between the couple and the MAP team.

11. Conclusion

I have argued here that criticisms of MAP ignore the fact that MAP may relieve the suffering of sterile couples. However, I have argued that this does not constitute a sufficient reason to give an ethical "blank cheque" to MAP, because MAP is a technology, and as such requires ethical discernment. Three ethical suggestions were made here: listen to those suffering from sterility, without necessarily endorsing everything they say; respect the complexity of the gift of life; and consider technical and scientific advances not as an end, but as a means to serve the couple's desire for a child (keeping resource constraints in mind). More ethical discussion of MAP is required.

12. References

Bydlowski, M. (2000a).*La dette de vie. Itinéraire psychanalytique de la maternité.* Paris: PUF, ISBN-10: 2130503535, ISBN-13: 978-2130503538, Paris.

Bydlowski, M. (2000b).*Je rêve un enfant. L'expérience intérieure de la maternité.* Paris: Odile Jacob, ISBN-10: 2738123996, ISBN-13: 978-2738123992, Paris.

Clerget, J. (2003). *"L'home devenant pere", in Le pere, l'homme et le masculin en perinatalite.* ed. P. Marciano P (Rarnonville Saint-Agne: Eres, 2003), ISBN 2-7492-0126-8.

Cohen, B.H. (2001).*Un bébé mais pas à tout prix. Les dessous de la médecine de la reproduction.* Paris: J.-C. Lattès, ISBN-10: 2290326682, ISBN-13: 978-2290326688.

Delaisi de Parseval, G & P. Verdier. (1994). *Enfant de personne.* Paris: Odile Jacob, France.

Delaisi de Parseval, G. (2003). *"Les PMA ou 'Paternites medicalement assistees", in Le pere, l'homrne et le masculin en perinatalite.* ed. P. Marciano P Ramonville Saint-Agne: Eres, ISBN 9782749201269.

Ellul, J. (1954).*La Technique ou L'Enjeu du siècle.* Paris: Armand Colin, 1954, Paris: Économica, 1990.

Flis-Trèves, M. (1998). *Elles veulent un enfant.* Paris: Albin Michel, ISBN 2226105441.

Fonty, B., & Hoguenin, J. (2003). *Les pères n'ont rien à faire dans les maternités* . Paris: Editions générales First, ISBN 2-87691-747-5, France.

Héritier, F. (1996). Masculin-Féminin. *La pensée de la différence* . Paris: Odile Jacob, 1996, ISBN 2-7381-1605-1, Paris.

Hermitte, M.H. (1990). *"L'embryon aléatoire", in Le magasin des enfants,* ed. J. Testart (Paris: François Bourin, 1990), 238-265.

Jéronymidès, E. (2001). *Elles aussi deviendront mères. Des femmes qui se sentent stériles.* Paris: Payot et Rivages, ISBN 2228893498 978 2228893497, France.

Koeppel, B. (2000). *La vie qui revient. Dans un service de fécondation in vitro.* Ed. Calmann-Lévy (10 mai 2000), ISBN-10: 2702131204, ISBN-13: 978-2702131206, France.

Malherbe,J.F. (1997). *Pour une éthique de la medicine.* Namur: Artel-Fides, ISBN 287374040X 9782873740405, Montreal, Canada.

Mehl, D. (1999). Naitre? : La controverse bioéthique . Paris: Bayard, 1999, ISBN 2227137738, ISBN 9782227137738.

Ravez, L. (2006).*Les amours auscultées: une nouvelle éthique pour l'assistance médicale à la procreation.* Paris: Les Ed. du Cerf, ISBN 2204079731 ISBN 9782204079730.

Roegiers, L. (2000). *Les cigognes en crise* (Bruxelles: De Boeck Université, 1994), ISBN 10: 2804119238, ISBN 13: 9782804119232 .4

6

Stem Cells: Ethical and Religious Issues

Farzaneh Zahedi-Anaraki and Bagher Larijani
Endocrinology and Metabolism Research Centre, Medical Ethics and History of Medicine Research Centre, Tehran University of Medical Sciences
Iran

1. Introduction

Stem cells are capable of generating various tissue cells which can be used for therapeutic approaches to debilitating and incurable disease. Even though many applications of stem cells are under investigation, such research has raised high hopes and promises along with warnings and ethical and religious questions in different societies. Generally, there is little concern about using non-human or adult stem cells. However, embryonic stem cell research has been confronted with questions from medical professionals, the public, religious groups, and national and international organizations. The debate is partly related to "personhood" and the notion of human dignity. Sources of stem cells, the moral status of human embryo, the slippery slope toward commercialisation of human life, concerns about safety, germ line intervention and the challenge of proportionality are some ethical issues.

Stem cell research is a promising but controversial issue on which many religions have taken strong positions. The point at which human life begins is a pivotal challenge. Conception, primitive streak development, implantation, ensoulment and birth are specific stages in which different groups claim dignity begins in the course of human development.

In this chapter, we will review the history and scientific facts of stem cells in brief; then, ethical considerations will be discussed. Our other aim is to clarify the religious debate on the issue, particularly monotheistic perspectives. Some related international and national guidelines will be reviewed in brief.

2. Definitions

In vivo (normal reproduction) or in vitro fertilization (IVF) of ova (female germ cells) and spermatozoa (male germ cells) forms *zygotes* which contain the total genetic materials, one half from the male DNA and one half from the female DNA. In favourable condition, the zygote divides and forms the *blastomere* (8 cells), and then the *blastocyst* (120-150 cells) around day five. Blastocysts consist of stem cells. At this stage, division of a blastocyst may produce two or more normal human embryos. During the third week of human development, the *primitive streak*, which is the primitive central nervous system, appears. At this stage, the embryo is a unique entity which is no longer twinnable. Some scientists consider this point as the moment when human life begins as such (Balint, 2001).

Stem cells in blastocysts are capable of differentiating along each of the germ layers of the ectoderm (skin, nerves, brain), the mesoderm (bone, muscle), and the endoderm (lungs, digestive system) (Hyun, 2008). After this stage of human foetus development, stem cells can be also found in different tissues but their capability is limited. For instance, as Lewis (2009) stated, while mesenchymal stem cells are able to produce bone, cartilage, and muscle, bone marrow stem cells can give rise only to white blood cells. The following part sheds more light on the issue.

3. Stem cells: The facts and promises

Stem cells are undifferentiated cells with the capacity of renewal which can be used for regeneration of body cells and tissues. Many potential therapeutic benefits are defined for different types of stem cells. Based on the power of differentiation, stem cells can be classified as totipotent, pluripotent, multipotent, and unipotent (table 1).

Term	Definition	Example	Sources
Totipotent	Able to produce an entire being	Blastomeres	Fertilized egg drived cells (1-3 days embryo)
Pluripotent	Able to differentiate to germ layers of ectoderm, mesoderm and endoderm	Embryonic stem cell	5-14 days embryo
Multi potent	Able to produce many cell types and self-renew over the lifetime of the being and over many subsequent generations if transplanted	Hematopoietic stem cell	Cord blood, fetal tissues, bone marrow, Adult stem cells
Unipotent	Able to differntiate to only one lineage, and with limited or no capacity of self-renewal	Neural stem cell	Adult stem cells
Induced pluripotent (iPS)	Normal adult cells reprogrammed to an embryonic state, able to produce all tissues	---	Derived from a non-pluripotent cell

Table 1. Stem cell classification and potential for differentiation.

Embryonic stem cells (ESCs) are able to produce all tissues and germ lines (sperm and eggs) and to self-renew indefinitely. These pluripotent stem cells were first isolated in 1998. However, the resources of ESCs are limited, and since human embryos have to be destroyed for ESC production, many people oppose the use of this kind of stem cell for scientific research or therapeutic approaches.

ESCs can be produced in the laboratory in two ways: by derivation from the inner cell mass (ICM) of a blastocyst in a 5-14 days embryo, or by somatic cell nuclear transfer (SCNT). SCNT or cloning, which was brought into public attention after cloning of the sheep "Dolly" in 1997 (Wilmut et al., 1997), is also used as a technique to produce stem cells for basic developmental biology research and cell-based therapies. Through cloning, the DNA of an unfertilized egg is replaced with the DNA of the patient's cell. Although a Korean scientist claimed to extract stem cells from human cloning in 2004 (Hwang, 2004, 2005), his work was recognized as a scientific fraud later on (Kennedy, 2006). Although there are important concerns about the safety of cloning, as Fischbach and Fischbach state, stem cells produced by therapeutic cloning have the advantage over those harvested from embryos resulting from IVF or aborted foetuses in that the cells generated through therapeutic cloning are genetically similar to the cells of the individual who donated the nucleus (Fischbach & Fischbach, 2004), therefore they are immunologically matched to the patient, which avoids problems of rejection (Coors, 2002; Weissman, 2002). Another source of pluripotent cells are human embryonic germ (hEG) cells which are derived from the gonadal ridges of aborted fetuses (Gogle et al., 2003; Balint, 2001).

Multipotent stem cells have a research history of more than 40 years and have been successfully used for treatment of some disorders such as leukaemia for decades (Hyne, 2008). The use of these stem cells is surrounded with less ethical and religious debate since they can be naturally found as adult stem cells throughout the body; however, their limited potential of differentiation has restricted their practical uses. Also, mass production of multipotent (and unipotent) stem cells is time consuming.

Inactive adult stem cells (SCs) exist in many tissues and need to be signalled. Haematopoietic SCs, which are used for bone marrow transplantation in oncology, are a good example of the use of this kind of SCs in cell and tissue transplantation. Medical waste, such as amniotic fluid, placenta, menstrual blood, synovial fluid from knee, teeth, liposuction aspirate, umbilical cords, is a source of adult stem cells (Lewis, 2009).

Induced pluripotent stem (iPS) cells have been reprogrammed with retroviruses to behave like embryonic stem cells (Hyne, 2008). The methods that reprogram adult human cells to a pluripotent state were described firstly by two groups of researchers from Japan and the United States (Takahashi et al., 2007; Blow, 2008). Considering the mutagenicity of the viruses and the potential to activate oncogenes, and the debate on their properties and potential as embryonic stem cells, iPS cells are not used as a practical therapeutic agent yet (Blow, 2008). Further experiments showed that reprogramming genes can be done in safer ways without the use of viruses (Lewis, 2009).

The main potential use of stem cells in medicine is for cell and tissue replacement therapies. There are hopes for lifelong treatment of disorders such as Huntington's disease, Parkinson's disease, type 1 diabetes mellitus, myocardial infarction, spinal cord injuries, stroke, chronic skin ulcers and burns by transplantation of stem cells. The utilization of stem cells in the treatment of Alzheimer's disease, avascular necrosis, neural deafness, osteoarthritis, liver failure, and some autoimmune disorders including multiple sclerosis (MS), rheumatoid arthritis, and systemic lupus erythematosus (SLE) is also under research.

Stem cell research may pave the way for designing novel approaches in regenerative medicine. Since ESCs can proliferate without limit and can differentiate to any cell type, they offer unprecedented access to tissues from the human body, and they have the potential to provide an unlimited amount of tissue for transplantation therapies to treat a wide range of degenerative diseases (National Institute of Health [NIH], 2006). Genetic research, understanding of normal development, research on the differentiation of human tissues, and birth defects investigations are other potential uses of stem cells. Stem cells can be used for drug development and toxicity tests too. They can support research on safety and efficacy of new drugs.

The therapeutic potential of stem cells has been publicized, and much related public enthusiasm has been reflected in some stories and movies. There are scientific, ethical, legal, religious, and social challenges for the use of stem cells for cell and tissue transplantation.

The concerns should be addressed before the widespread use of this science and technology. We intend to review main ethical issues and religious perspectives in the following sections.

4. Ethical issues

Moral arguments for and against stem cell research and therapy are many, regarding issues such as the types of cells, the sources and techniques of production, and utilization. There are few concerns about research on or therapeutic uses of adult stem cells. But embryonic stem cells have been associated with serious ethical debates. The use of this new science and technology for human reproduction has triggered ethics and policy disputes around the world. Human cloning has been a cause of concern for ethicists, lawyers, religious scholars, sociologists and politicians, among others.

There are different challenges in different societies. The study by Zarzeczny and Caulfield (2009) confirms the complexity of the issues raised by stem cell research. The results of this study, which was carried out in Canada, suggest some main themes, including: theories/views on policy development, issues with focus on science and health, issues related to the supply of embryos, debates on novel technologies such as cloning, non-embryonic sources of stem cells, jurisdictional competition, intellectual property issues, the need for guidelines and standards, research funding issues, and stem cell tourism (Zarzeczny & Caulfield, 2009).

Related ethical issues may be discussed using different ethical approaches, such as utilitarianism, deontology, and principlism. Each approach may justify or reject the use of stem cells in research or therapeutics. For instance, according to the utilitarian approach, the consequences of stem cell utilization should be assessed using the benefit to harm ratio as a measure to accept or reject the new technology. In a deontologic (duty-based) approach, the duty to help those who suffer or to save lives may permit research or therapy with stem cells. In principle-based ethics, various principles should be discussed collectively to evaluate the rightness or wrongness of use of stem cells.

People who oppose or support stem cell research can be philosophically divided into different categories. For instance, some opponents emphasize the dignity of human beings and that every person is an end and not only a means to some other end. This idea is consistent with deontology. It means that every person, likely including a foetus, should be respected and protected (balint, 2001). On the other hand, those who support research on human stem cells, either in religious or secular bioethics, support the advantages of such research to save human lives and the duty to relieve suffering in accordance with utilitarian and duty-based approaches. Some even go so far as to state that such research is a "moral imperative", considering the potential benefits of ameliorating human suffering (Balint, 2001).

There are important issues, such as respect for human dignity, which may influence these discussions. Ethical issues will be discussed in the following without reference to the philosophic basis.

4.1 Human dignity

In the process of stem cell research, stem cells must be extracted from the blastocyst, so the human embryo is destroyed. Opponents of stem cell research claim that the destruction of human embryos is morally equivalent to the killing of a human being.

The morality of destroying human embryos for the benefit of others is the main argument in both secular and religious bioethics. Opinions regarding the ontological status of preimplantation embryos vary widely. Some hold the "conceptionalist" view, according to which the embryo is a "person", considering its potential to develop into a person. Others believe that the embryo (and even the fetus) is a "non-person", and that it ought not to be attributed much, if any, moral status (DeWert & Mummery, 2003).

There is another viewpoint of the "relative value" of human embryos, more than cells but less than persons (Hinman, 2009). This view states that embryos deserve respect but not to the same extent as a fully developed person. According to this moral argument, the moral status of a human embryo gradually increases through its development in the uterus, and at the point of birth it is entitled to enjoy full rights of human beings (United Nations Educational, Scientific and Cultural Organization, 2004).

Another moral argument states that the status of embryos differs across milestones in the process of embryonic development (United Nations Educational, Scientific and Cultural Organization, 2004). In this argument, the question is at what point after fertilization of egg by sperm the cell mass becomes a human being. This seems an ethical impasse which science may not be able to resolve. For ethical decision making on stem cell research, we should determine when a new human entity comes into existence. According to the scientific facts, there are significant points for delineation of human embryos, including: the moment of fertilization, the point of implantation in the uterus, the initial appearance of the primitive streak (19 days), the beginning of heartbeat (23 days), the development of brain waves (48 days), the point at which essential internal and external structures are complete (56 days), the point at which the fetus begins to move (12-13 weeks) (Hinman, 2009), and the point when the foetus would be viable outside the uterus (Balint, 2001).

As mentioned above, during the third week of human embryo development, the primitive streak develops and three germ layers appear. Before this stage, embryos can split and produce two or more embryos; however, after development of the primitive streak, the embryo is a unique entity. In view of this fact, many believe that ontological individuality starts at this point, hence the embryo can be used for research prior to this stage; up to 14 days of development (DeWert & Mummery, 2003).

Religious schools also make various points which will be discussed later. There is no doubt that an embryo is a living being whether or not it merits human rights. However, an entity would have the full rights and privileges of human beings when personhood begins.

There are different views on preimplantation embryos. Some bioethicists suggested "the trajectory argument" to defend the human rights of a human embryo before implantation (Hinman, 2009). According to this argument, since an early embryo has the potential to be a human being in the future, it deserves protection. However, others claim that an entity before implantation is no more than a seed. There is also another viewpoint, according to which human embryos, even if they are not persons, deserve respect (Hinman, 2009). As Hinman (2009, slide 20) concludes: "*We can see some advocates of both sides of the hESCdebate as accepting the general principle of respect for innocent human life; their disagreement may not be over the principle, but over the way in which the principle is to be applied in particular cases.*"

The fear of "instrumentalization" of human embryos is a barrier to create embryos (DeWert & Mummery, 2003). However, despite opposition to creation of embryos for research, there are arguments in support of the use of spare embryos in the process of IVF as sources of embryonic stem cells because such embryos would be destroyed anyway. Several hundred thousands of unwanted embryos are discarded annually in IVF clinics. The use of such embryos before the appearance of the primitive streak is supported by many ethicists.

However, as stem cells that are derived from surplus embryos may cause immune rejection when transplanted to a patient, some researchers emphasize the production of genetically identical stem cells by the use of cloning or other techniques in order to avoid immune rejection in transplantation (United Nations Educational, Scientific and Cultural Organization, 2004).

The research carried out in Canada (Zarzeczny & Caulfield, 2009) shows that even though issues related to the moral status of embryos continue to be a main issue in the literature on stem cell research, discourses associated with the moral status of embryos may not receive the same attention in social and other realms. For instance, while the moral status of embryos has a central role in legal discourse, it plays a relatively minor role in print media (Zarzeczny & Caulfield, 2009).

4.2 Safety

Many people are excited about the potential benefits of stem cells in clinical practice. There are many claims about the power of stem cells as an unparalleled cure in medicine. Potential benefits coupled with great public interest have produced significant pressures on scientists to continue research. Along with the promises, stem cell science poses a threat to human safety. As Dresser (2010) states, many claims about the therapeutic power of stem cells lack a solid evidentiary foundation and many data are not examined in human clinical trials. In other words, there is much to learn regarding the use of stem cells for the treatment of diseases. Therefore, prior to any decision about using stem cells, their safety and efficacy must be determined.

Risks of stem cell treatment, including tumors after stem cell injections (Amariglio et al., 2009, as cited in Lindvall, et al., 2004, 2006), drew attention to safety issues and importance of medical and ethical standards before clinical application of this new type of treatment. Some who agree with stem cell research claim that such research is still in the early stages and very far from clinical, therapeutic or reproductive uses.

Based on the principle of non-maleficence, harms to the embryo cannot be justified by future benefits to society. It is also suggested that "... *the harm done to the society by allowing the destruction of embryos is more significant.*" (Balint, 2001).

4.3 Informed consent

Many scientists believe that people are misinformed about stem cells, their sources, their potential benefits, and harms. It also seems that medical companies and industries are optimistic about stem cell future. So, a demand for stem cell research and therapy has been created in many societies. Some centres for the treatment are in countries with a lesser ethical oversight, such as China and some Eastern European countries. An increase in stem cell tourism has received attention in many countries (Zarzeczny, 2010). For these reasons, disclosure of information to patients and their families is essential. Murdoch et al (2010, page 21) have emphasized that such disclosure should have at least three elements:

"*1. Disclose and discuss the potential for real physical, psychological, and economic harm from the interventions and travel, including costs of the procedure relative to patient's means.*

2. Disclose and relay independent scientific evidence of risk or benefit for a defined intervention.

3. Disclose any evidence of ethical misconduct or questionable practices. This includes:

- *Failure to supply local and national evidence of oversight.*
- *Engaging in questionable patient recruiting practices.*

- *Clear misrepresentation, fraud, or patient abuse.*"

As mentioned before, the extra embryos of IVF clinics which are no longer wanted by the parents are sources for stem cell research. Obtaining consent for such embryos is problematic. There are questions of whether consent of biological parents is enough and how the consent should be obtained and recorded. Also, as Balint (2001) states, there may be emotional pressure on parents to consent. The parents' feelings and beliefs may also cause additional anxiety and a sense of guilt about embryo donation for use in research.

Consent of gamete donors in cases of IVF should also be obtained and recorded. Many ethicists are worried about risks to women who participate in the egg production process. In the Korean cloning fraud, one ethical problem was related to the egg collection from the subordinate women staff, which raised the issue of coercion and violation of their rights (Longstaff et al., 2009, as cited in Saunders & Savulescu, 2008). From a feminist perspective, the instrumental use of women in the process of the creation of embryos for research is an important concern, since the creation of human embryos for research purposes requires the harvesting of eggs from women (United Nations Educational, Scientific and Cultural Organization, 2004). In animal cloning, there is a need for hundreds of unfertilized eggs to produce one cloned embryo. In women, there has to be a period of hormone treatment followed by invasive surgery to obtain oocytes for research purposes. In addition to the risk of exploitation of women and commercialization of human eggs (United Nations Educational, Scientific and Cultural Organization, 2004), there may be life-threatening risks such as Ovarian Hyper-stimulation Syndrome (OHSS).

4.4 Slippery slope

A slippery slope argument is used by opponents of stem cell research, who cast doubt on the morality of the use of stem cells by reasoning that if we accept the creation and destroying of human embryos in the process of such research, there is no logical cut-off point by which we can distinguish the point at which destroying a human embryo is permissible. As Evers (2002) states, it may open the way to a slippery slope of dehumanizing practices, such as embryo farms, cloned babies, the use of fetuses for spare parts, and the commodification of human life.

The right to reproductive freedom in individualistic social systems may be used to justify reproductive approaches with use of stem cells. Some opponents claim that eradication of an entity like a human zygote is similar to abortion, which thus has a link to stem cell research (Dresser, 2010). All societies should take a stand on the issue of eradication of human embryos in the process of stem cell research.

4.5 Resource allocation and commercialization

There are many patients, scientists, politicians and even bioethicists who have paid tribute to stem cell therapy and its hypes and hopes (Murdoch, et al., 2010), despite debates on safety and efficacy. Commodification of human embryos is a concern expressed by many ethicists. There may be loss of equity in access to stem cell benefits, as many people would not be able to pay the high cost of this new treatment.

Resource allocation and distributive justice are related important issues. Limited resources of health care systems raise questions about research priorities in many societies. Stem cell research is expensive, and its outcome may not be useful for many patients or healthy people. Thus, it could be argued that money can be more effectively spent for more important health care plans which cover a vast range of diseases and large numbers of the general population.

However, many argue that banning stem cell research by governments would not stop such research in the private sector. Private research can raise concerns about commercialization of stem cell research, which may result in unfair distribution of benefits within society (Balint, 2001). So, some conclude that federal funding and support of research on embryonic stem cells is the only approach that may guarantee the fair distribution of benefits (Balint, 2001). Moreover, such policy can provide the way for more strict observance of ethical standards by researchers.

Private sectors usually tend to allocate their resources to fields with high potential of financial gain. However, priority of resource allocation in the public budget by governments depends on some other factors, including: public health needs, scientific value of the proposal, potential for advances in a particular area, distribution across diverse research areas, and national training and infrastructure needs (Dresser, 2010). Funding stem cell research is not considered a research priority in some countries, due to other health care needs and limitations of health budget. Many underdeveloped or developing countries are obligated to devote research funds to common disorders with high rates of mortality and morbidity.

Stem cell tourism and fear of negative health consequences due to lack of enough oversight are other concerns which have attracted special attention among ethicists and medical practitioners. Such matters deserve separate discussion elsewhere, particularly as they are not unique to stem cells.

4.6 Other issues

Many ethical issues associated with the use of stem cells apply to biomedical research generally. Some issues which were discussed above, such as priorities of research and allocation of limited resources, disclosure of truth about benefits and harms, and obtaining consent, are prominent in stem cell research. Paying appropriate attention to research integrity and related matters such as responsible conduct of research, ownership of data, and authorship, are particularly emphasized in this field.

Another relevant general ethical issue is that of conflict of interests. There are financial interests for researchers who work in this field. Honesty and openness of researchers, along with appropriate independent review of research, are required.

Some issues are more specific and require special attention. For instance, stem cells can be used for the study of normal development of human embryos and for genetic research. Therefore, concerns about germ lines interventions attempting eugenics have been raised (Balint, 2001).

An issue is the principle of subsidiarity, according to which stem cell research can be ethically permissible only if there are no alternatives (DeWert & Mummery, 2003). Some options have been discussed as alternatives of human embryonic stem cells, which consist of: human embryonic germ (hEG) cells, adult stem cells, and xenotransplantation. For comparison of these alternatives, many elements should be analysed, including: burdens and/or risks, the chance of success and applicability, and the time-scale in which clinically useful applications are to be expected (DeWert & Mummery, 2003). Low success rates of the use of hEG cells and uncertain outcomes, and cross-species infections caused by xenotransplantation and high rates of immunity rejection are the barriers for the first and third alternatives.

Adult stem cells experiments have had great success in recent decades. Scientists have been studying them since the 1960s (United Nations Educational, Scientific and Cultural Organization, 2004). Avoidance of immunity system rejection problems is an important advantage of these cells. However, there are many doubts about their developmental potential and their proliferation capacity as a substitute for embryonic stem cells (Kuehnle & Goodell, 2002; Gavaghan, 2001).

As mentioned above, iPS cells are suggested as another alternative for human embryonic stem cells (Hyne, 2008; Takahashi et al., 2007; Blow, 2008). Many experiments have been done in recent years to test the efficacy and safety of this novel option (Lewis, 2009).

Aborted foetuses are suggested as sources for obtaining germ line stem cells, though critical issues are raised (Balint, 2001). Women coercion, their safety, stem cell recipient safety, informed consent issues, and vulnerability of the foetus are concerns which cause this suggestion to remain controversial.

According to some advocates, stem cell research can save many lives. But the principle of proportionality urges ethicists to weigh potential benefits and harms. Pursuance of medical progress at any cost does not seem ethical.

5. Legislation and guidelines

During recent decades, stem cell research has posed a challenge for politicians and national and international regulatory agencies. Despite challenges across different societies, stem cell research continues to be conducted by researchers. The need for oversight and regulation to prevent unethical conduct and negative outcomes is recognized by many scientists. As a result, international and national bodies have tried to guide stem cell activities ethically.

General ethical guidelines such as the Belmont report (Department of Health, Education, and Welfare, 1979), Helsinki declaration (The World Medical Association [WMA], 2008), and International Ethical Guidelines for Biomedical Research Involving Human Subjects (Council for International Organizations of Medical Sciences [CIOMS], 2002) should be observed by stem cell researchers. There are also specific stem cell guidelines and standards internationally and in various countries.

Establishment of international ethical guidelines and legal frameworks for human cloning was considered at the end of the 20th century. The issue of reproductive cloning was discussed several times in United Nations agencies after the birth of Dolly in 1997. In 1998, the United Nations General Assembly endorsed a Declaration in which reproductive cloning of human beings was banned (United Nations Educational, Scientific and Cultural Organization, 2004).

The Universal Declaration on the Human Genome and Human Rights (The United Nations Educational, Scientific and Cultural Organization [UNESCO], 1997) (Section C-Article 11), and the report of UNESCO's International Bioethics Committee (IBC) on "The Use of Embryonic Stem Cells in Therapeutic Research" (UNESCO, 2001) were compiled to address these complex issues in different societies. Other international organizations such as the World Health Organization (WHO) compiled relevant resolutions too.

The International Society for Stem Cell Research (ISSCR) has also tried to address relevant scientific, cultural, religious, ethical, and legal differences across national borders by preparation of the "Guidelines for the Conduct of Human Embryonic Stem Cell Research" (ISSCR, 2006). The mission of the taskforce for compiling the guidelines was stated as: "*...to emphasize the responsibility of scientists to ensure that human stem cell research is carried out* *according to rigorous standards of research ethics, and to encourage uniform research practices that should be followed by all human stem cell scientists globally.*" Due to the ever-increasing therapeutic uses of stem cells in clinical practice, the "Guidelines for the Clinical Translation of Stem Cells", were compiled in 2008 (ISSCR, 2008). The Guidelines address three major areas of translational stem cell research: (a) cell processing and manufacture; (b) preclinical studies; and (c) clinical research.

As to the disputes on the time when personhood starts, the guidelines and Acts determine this. The United Kingdom's Human Fertilization and Embryology Act, for instance, determines the point of primitive streak development as the point when human life begins and research must be stopped (Balint, 2001, citation of Human Fertilization and Embryology Act, 1990).

As Childress (2004) emphasizes, the connection between ethics and public policy remains important. Two types of public policies have special relevance to human stem cell research, public policies on use of governmental funds, and public policies on whether, apart from the use of governmental funds, to permit, regulate, or prohibit activities such as human cloning (Childress, 2004).

Many societies have attempted to characterize the legal status of the human embryo and regulate stem cell research. Considerable differences exist between countries in the regulation of stem cell research. In the United states, the National Bioethics Advisory Committee (NBAC) decided that creation of embryos purely for research purposes was not acceptable, while in the United Kingdom, the Human Fertilization and embryology Authority permits the creation of embryos for research but the embryos must never be implanted (Balint, 2001). In addition, in the United Kingdom and some other countries where stem cell research under national regulations is permitted, there are standard guidelines and recommendations for public and private sectors; there are no such regulations and supervision in the US (Balint, 2001). The National Institutes of Health (NIH) provided guidelines on Human stem cell research with the aim of "*Removing Barriers to Responsible Scientific Research Involving Human Stem Cells*" (NIH, 2009).

In Canada, *Human Pluripotent Stem Cell Research Guidelines* released by the Canadian Institutes of Health Research (Canadian Institutes of Health Research, 2010), and the Assisted Human Reproductive Act (Health Canada, 2004), are the most important regulations concerning the use of stem cells in research and reproductive technologies.

In Costa Rica and Germany, eradication of embryos for research purposes is prohibited. Some countries, such as Belgium and the United Kingdom, allow research on surplus embryos and created embryos within 14 days after fertilization. In Denmark and Japan, while research on surplus embryos is permissible, the creation of embryos solely for research purposes is prohibited (United Nations Educational, Scientific and Cultural Organization, 2004). Many European countries have prohibited reproductive cloning, but there is a wide spectrum of diverse religious and secular beliefs about that (Nippert, 2002).

In the Middle East, Iran, as a pioneer country in stem cell research (Ilkilic and Ertin, 2010; Saniei and De Vries, 2008) that reported the establishment of a new stem cell line in 2003 (Baharvand et al, 2004), has recently established ethical guidelines for stem cell research and treatments in the country (Nejad-Sarvari et al, 2011).

Banning public funding for stem cell research in some countries like the US caused some worry about potential "brain drain", but funding the research costs by non-profit and private sectors has offered many opportunities for scientists to follow such research in these countries (Dresser, 2010).

6. Religious perspectives

As mentioned before, determination of the moment at which human life begins is pivotal in stem cell debates. Ensoulment is defined as the time when the entity becomes a human being, based on many religions' perspectives, although the moment when the soul arrives is long disputed.

Judaism considers the extracorporeal embryo in the preimplantation stage as genetic material, so stem cell research is permissible according to most branches of Judaism (Hinman, 2009; Childress, 2004; Ohara, 2003; Bioethics Advisory commission, 2000). A human embryo is not considered as sacred until the fourth month of pregnancy, according to most Jewish scholars (Pompe et al, 2005). Owing to this fact, research on stem cell and human embryos is allowed in this period.

In Christianity, while the current dominant belief is that ensoulment occurs at the moment of conception, the Roman Catholic theologian, Thomas Aquinas, believed that the soul arrives around the third month of pregnancy (quickening). St. Augustine believed that personhood begins with ensoulment at forty days of gestation, in accordance with Aristotle's and Talmudic scholars' views (Balint, 2001). Although this opinion was accepted by Popes innocent III (1211 AD) and Gregory XIII (1550 AD), increased use of abortion in the 18th century led to a change in the Church's thinking. As a result, Pope Pius IX decreed that ensoulment occurs at fertilization, and his viewpoint was followed by the Orthodox Church (Balint, 2001).

Currently, the Catholic Church believes personhood begins at conception (Daar et al., 2004). Despite strong opposition of Catholics to stem cell research, Protestants have a wider range of views (Childress, 2004; Ohara, 2003; Bioethics Advisory commission, 2000). Less conservative Protestant Christians support stem cell research at least before the development of the primitive streak at 14 days after fertilization (Fadel, 2007).

Most Muslim thinkers accept embryonic stem cell research (Childress, 2004; Ohara, 2003; Bioethics Advisory commission, 2000), although there are obstacles to the research in some Islamic countries (Ilkilic & Ertin, 2010). According to Islamic teachings, decisions on stem cell research and cloning research should be based on advantages and limitations. Considering inevitable consequences of reproductive cloning, it is prohibited by many Muslim religious authorities; however, stem cell research and cloning for therapeutic purposes is sometimes permissible with precautions in pre-ensoulment stages of fetus development (Larijani & Zahedi, 2004). Most branches of Islam consider ensoulment as the moment when the entity would have a full value of human beings, though the moral singularity of humans occurs at implantation.

Holy Quran depicts the different stages of human development in the womb in verses 12-14 of the chapter (Sura) of Al-Mumenoon (the Believers). Based on these verses and some other Islamic resources, it is accepted by Muslim scholars that ensoulment takes place at 120 days after conception (Aksoy, 2005; Morrison and Khademhosseini, 2011). It is noteworthy that in Islam human embryonic life is entitled to respect at any stages even before the breathing of spirit into the fetus (Fadel, 2007); however, the respect grows as the weeks pass until ensoulment when the child deserves the full respect of human being. As Ilkilic and Ertin (2010) state "...the ensoulment gives the embryo an exceptional moral status, which is decisive for the ethical assessment of any medical intervention affecting the embryo." So, experimental activities and therapeutic uses of stem cells are permissible before ensoulment with necessary precautions when they are justifiable based on Islamic principles such as the public interest. Looking for scientific advancements and seeking new treatments for human disorders may also apply to justify the use of human embryonic stem cells (Fadel, 2007).

The source of stem cells has been considered by Islamic scholars in issuing fatwa (religious decree) on permissibility of stem cell research. For instance, the scholars in the confereence of the Muslim World League's Islamic Jurisprudence Council held in Mecca in 2003 issued that the use of stem cells for therapy or scientific research is permitted as long as the cells' sources are permissible. Adults who consent, placenta or umbilical cord blood, excess fertilized eggs produced during the course of IVF and spontaneously aborted embryos are some acceptable resources, and intentionally aborted fetuses are forbidden to be used as a source for stem cells (Fadel, 2007, citation of Muslim Word League, 2003).

7. Conclusion

Human stem cells have introduced many hopes in medicine. There are still many scientific questions and unknowns surrounding the issue. Stem cell therapeutic options may not have widespread application in the short term. Significant concerns exist about the ethical, social and legal consequences of the use of the cells in research and treatment. Bioethicists, religious leaders, regulatory bodies, and political bodies have discussed these matters and attempted to address the consequences in appropriate ways. We aimed to review some relevant challenges in this chapter, in the hope of strengthening the relation between science and ethics. The various positions that different monotheistic religions have adopted regarding this novel type of research were also reviewed in this chapter.

Stem cell science is rapidly evolving in the world; however, finding alternatives and carrying out parallel research are important. While some scientists believe that ethical concerns are barriers to scientific progress, others are worried about the harms and seek new alternatives such as iPS cells which can address the issue of human dignity in the field of stem cell research.

Given the promises of stem cell research, it seems that there is a conflict between the duty to reduce suffering and the duty to respect human life. It is more sensible to regulate stem cell research than to ban it. In countries with government-sponsored activities in the field of stem cell research, ethical observance and control over private and public activities can be more effectively maintained.

Stem cell markets and tourism should be controlled, regulated and supervised. The general public should be engaged more actively in this discussion and in finding solutions and guidelines.

8. References

Aksoy, S. (2005). Making regulations and drawing up legislation in Islamic countries under conditions of uncertainty, with special reference to embryonic stem cell research. Journal of Medical Ethics, Vol. 31, No. 7, pp. 399-403, ISSN 0306-6800, eISSN 1473 4257.

Amariglio, N; Hirshberg, A; Scheithauer, BW; Cohen, Y; Loewenthal, R; Trakhtenbrot, L., et al. (2009). Donor-derived brain tumor following neural stem cell transplantation in an ataxia telangiectasia patient. *PLoS Med*, Vol. 6, No. 2, (February 2009), e1000029, pp. 0221-0231, ISSN 1549-1277, eISSN 1549-1676.

Baharvand, H; Ashtiani, SK; Valojerdi, MR; Shahverdi, A; Taee, A; Sabour, D. (2004). Establishment and in vitro differentiation of a new embryonic stem cell line from human blastocyst. *Differentiation*, Vol. 72, no. 5, (Jun 2004), pp. 224-9, ISSN 0301 4681, eISSN 1432-0436.

Balint JA. (2001). Ethical issues in stem cell research. In: Ethics and Law in stem cell research Panel, Date of access: February 25, 2011, Available from: <http://www.albanylawreview.org/archives/65/3/EthicalIssuesinStemCellResearch.pdf >

Bioethics Advisory commission. (2000). Summary of presentations on religious perspectives relating to research involving human stem cells, 1999. In: *Ethical issues in human stem cell research*. Vol. 1, Bioethics Advisory commission, Rockville, June 2000, pp. 99-104.

Blow, N. (2008). Stem Cells: A new path to pluripotency. *Nature*, Vol. 451, No. 7180, (13 February 2008), pp. 858-858, ISSN 00280836, eISSN 1476-4687.

Canadian Institutes of Health Research. (2010). Updated Guidelines for Human Pluripotent Stem Cell Research, June 30, 2010. Retrieved from <http://www.cihr-irsc.gc.ca/e/42071.html >

Childress, JF. (2004). Human stem cell research: some controversies in bioethics and public policy. *Blood Cells, Molecules, and Diseases*, Vol.32, (January-February 2004), pp. 100-105, ISSN 1079-9796.

Coors ME. (2002). Therapeutic cloning: from consequences to contradiction. *Journal of Medicine and Philosophy*, Vol.27, No.3, 2002. pp. 297-317, ISSN 0360-5310, eISSN 1744-5019.

Council for International Organizations of Medical Sciences (CIOMS). (2002). International Ethical Guidelines for Biomedical Research Involving Human Subjects. Available from: < http://www.cioms.ch/publications/layout_guide2002.pdf >

Daar, AS; Court, BE; Singer, PA. (2004). Stem cell research and transplantation: science leading ethics. *Transplant Proceedings*, Vol.36, No.8, (Oct 2004), pp. 2504-2506, ISSN 0041-1345.

Department of Health, Education, and Welfare. (1979). The Belmont report. Available from: < http://ohsr.od.nih.gov/guidelines/belmont.html>

DeWert, G; Mummery, CH. (2003). Human embryonic stem cells: research, ethics and policy. Human Reproduction, Vol.18, No.4, (April 2003), pp. 672-682, eISSN 1460-2350 , ISSN 0268-1161.

Dresser, R. (2010). Stem cell research as innovation: Expanding the Ethical and Policy Conversation. *The Journal of Law, Medicine & Ethics*, Vol. 38, No. 2, pp. 332–341, (Summer 2010), eISSN 1748 -720X.

Evers K. (2002). European perspectives on therapeutic cloning. *The New England Journal of Medicine*, Vol.346, No.20, (May 16, 2002), pp. 1579-82, ISSN 0028-4793, eISSN 1533-4406.

Fadel, HE. (2007). Prospects and Ethics of Stem Cell Research: An Islamic Perspective. *Journal of the Islamic Medical Association of North America* (JIMA), Vol. 39, No. 2, pp. 73-83, ISSN 0899- 8299, eISSN 2160-9829.

Fischbach, GD; Fischbach RL. (2004). Stem cells: science, policy, and ethics. *The Journal of Clinical Investigation*, Vol.14, No.10, (Nov 15, 2004), pp. 1364-1370, ISSN 0021-9738, eISSN 1558-8238.

Gavaghan, H. (2001). The promise of stem cells. *Bulletin of the world Health Organization*, Vol.79, No.8, (2001), pp. 800-801, ISSN 0042 9686.

Gogle, CR; Guthrie, SM; Sanders, RC; Allen, WL; Scott, EW; Peterson, BE. (2003). An overview of stem cell research and regulatory issues. *Mayo Clinic Proceedings*, Vol.78, (August 2003), pp. 993-1003, ISSN 0025-6196, eISSN 1942-5546.

Health Canada. (2004). Assisted Human Reproduction Act (AHRA). Retrieved from: <http://laws-lois.justice.gc.ca/eng/acts/A-13.4/FullText.html >

Hinman LM. (2009). The Ethics of Stem Cell Research. In: *Lectures in Applied Ethics*, Date of access: March 27, 2011, Available from: <http://ethics.sandiego.edu/Presentations/AppliedEthics/StemCellEthics/StemCellEthics.pdf>

Hwang, WS; Roh, SI; Lee, BC; Kang, SK; Kwon, DK; Kim, S; et al. (2005). Patient-Specific Embryonic Stem Cells Derived from Human SCNT Blastocysts. *Science*, Vol. 308, No. 5729, pp.1777-83, ISSN 0036-8075, eISSN 1095-9203.

Huwang, WS; Ryu, YJ; Park, JH; Park, ES; Lee, EG; Koo, JM; et al. (2004). Evidence of a pluripotent human embryonic stem cell line derived from a cloned blastocysts. *Science*, Vol. 303, No.5664, 2004, pp. 1669-1674, ISSN 0036 8075, eISSN 1095 9203

Hyun, I. (2008). Stem Cells, In: *From Birth to Death and Bench to Clinic: The Hastings Center Bioethics Briefing Book for Journalists, Policymakers, and Campaigns*, Mary Crowley (ed.), pp. 159-162, The Hastings Center, Retrieved from: < http://www.thehastingscenter.org/Publications/BriefingBook/>

Ilkilic, I; Ertin, H. (2010). Ethical aspects of human embryonic stem cell research in the islamic world: positions and reflections. *Stem Cell Rev*, Vol. 6, No. 2, (June 2010), pp.151-61, ISSN 1550 -8943.

International Society for Stem Cell Research (ISSCR). (2006). Guidelines for the Conduct of Human Embryonic Stem Cell Research. ISSCR, Retrieved from < http://www.isscr.org/guidelines/ISSCRhESCguidelines2006.pdf >

International Society for Stem Cell Research (ISSCR). (2008). Guidelines for the Clinical Translation of Stem Cells. ISSCR, Retrieved from: < http://www.isscr.org/clinical_trans/pdfs/ISSCRGLClinicalTrans.pdf >

Kennedy, D. (2006). Editorial Retraction. *Science*, Vol. 335, No. 5759, pp. 335, ISSN 0036- 8075 eISSN 1095- 9203.

Kuehnle, L; Goodell, MA. (2002). The therapeutic potential of stem cells from adults. *BMJ*, Vol.325, (Augest 2002), pp. 372-376, ISSN 1759 2151.

Larijani, B; Zahedi, F. (2004). Islamic perspective on human cloning and stem cell research. *Transplantation Proceedings*, Vol.36, No.10, (Dec 2004), pp. 3188- 3189, ISSN 0041 1345.

Lewis, R. (2009). A stem cell primer. *Biology Digest*, Vol. 35, No. 9, pp. 11-19, (May 2009), ISSN: 0095-2958.

Longstaff, H; Schuppli, CA; Preto, N; Lafrenière, D; McDonald, M. (2009). Scientists' Perspectives on the Ethical Issues of Stem Cell Research. *Stem Cell Rev and Rep*, Vol. 5, No. 2, (June 2009), pp. 89–95, ISSN 1550-8943, eISSN 1558-6804.

Morrison, DWG; Khademhosseini, A. (access 2011). Stem Cell Science in Iran. Published by the Iranian Studies Group (ISG) at Massachusetts Institute of Technology (MIT). Available from: <http://isgmit.org/projects-storage/StemCell/stem_cell_iran.pdf>

Murdoch, CE; Scott, CT. (2010). Stem Cell Tourism and the Power of Hope, *The American Journal of Bioethics*, Vol. 10, No. 5, (May 2010), pp.16-23, ISSN 1526-5161, eISSN 1536-0075 .

National Institute of Health [NIH]. (2006). *Regenerative medicine* 2006, Retrieved from <http://stemcells.nih.gov/staticresources/info/scireport/PDFs/Regenerative_Medicine_2006.pdf >

National Institutes of Health (NIH). (2009). NIH Guidelines for Human Stem Cell Research. Retrieved from < http://stemcells.nih.gov/policy/2009guidelines.htm >

Nejad-sarvari, N; Emami-razavi, SH; Larijani, B; Zahedi, F. (2011). The proposal of ethical guidelines in stem cell research and treatments in Iran. *Journal of Medical Ethics and History of Medicine*, vol. 4, No. 2, pp. 15-24, eISSN: 2008-0387. Available from: < http://journals.tums.ac.ir/upload_files/pdf/17809.pdf> (in Farsi)

Nippert, I. (2002). The pros and cons of human therapeutic cloning in the public debate. J Biotechnol , Vol.98, No.1, (Sep 2002), pp. 53-60, ISSN 0168 -1656.

Ohara, N. (2003). Ethical consideration of experimentation using living human embryo: the Catholic Church's position on human embryonic stem cell research and human cloning. *Clin Exp Obstet Gynecol*, Vol.30, No.2-3, 2003, pp. 77–81, ISSN 0390-6663.

Pompe, S; Bader, M; Tannert, Christof. (2005). Stem-cell research: the state of the art. *EMBO Reports*, Vol. 6, No. 4, (April 2005), pp. 297–300, ISSN 1469 221X.

Saniei M, De Vries R. (2008). Embryonic stem cell research in Iran: status and ethics. *Indian J Med Ethics*, Vol. 5, No. 4, Oct-Dec 2008, pp. 181-4, ISSN 0974-8466.

Takahashi, K; Tanabe, K; Ohnuki, M; Narita, M; Ichisaka, T; Tomoda, K; Yamanaka, SH. (2007). Induction of Pluripotent Stem Cells from Adult Human Fibroblasts by Defined Factors. *Cell*, Vol. 131, No. 5, pp. 861-72, ISSN 0092-8674.

The United Nations Educational, Scientific and Cultural Organization (UNESCO). (1997). The Universal Declaration on the Human Genome and Human Rights. Available from: <http://www.unesco.org/new/en/social-and-human-sciences/themes/bioethics/human-genome-and-human-rights/>

The United Nations Educational, Scientific and Cultural Organization (UNESCO). (2001). The Use of Embryonic Stem Cells in Therapeutic Research. Available from: < http://www.eubios.info/UNESCO/ibc2001sc.pdf >

The World Medical Association (WMA). (2008). Declaration of Helsinki. Available from: < http://www.wma.net/en/30publications/10policies/b3/17c.pdf>

United Nations Educational, Scientific and Cultural Organization. (2004). Human cloning: ethical issues. France: UNESCO, SHS-2004. Retrieved from: < http://unesdoc.unesco.org/images/0013/001359/135928e.pdf >

Weissman IL. (2002). Stem cells-scientific, medical and political issues. *The New England Journal of Medicine*, Vol.346, No.20, 2002, pp. 1576-1579, ISSN 0028-4793, eISSN 1533 - 4406.

Wilmut, I; Schnieke, AE; McWhir, J; Kind, AJ; Campbell, KHS. (1997). Viable offspring derived from fetal and adult mammalian cells. *Nature*, Vol. 385, No. 6619, pp. 810-13, (27 February 1997), ISSN 0028- 0836, eISSN 1476 -4687.

Zarzeczny, A; Caulfield, T. (2009). Emerging Ethical, Legal and Social Issues Associated with Stem Cell Research & and the Current Role of the Moral Status of the Embryo.

Stem Cell Rev and Rep, Vol. 5, No.2, (June 2009), pp. 96-1ffi, ISSN 155-8943 eISSN 1558-6804.

Zarzeczny, A; Caulfield, T. (2010). Stem Cell Tourism and Doctors 1 Duties to Minors-A View From Canada, The *American Journal of Bioethics,* Vol. 10, No.5, (May 2010), pp.3-15, ISSN 1526-5161, eISSN1536-0075.

7

The "Cultural Differences" Argument and Its Misconceptions: The Return of Medical Truth-Telling in China

Jing-Bao Nie
[1]University of Otago
[2](Adjunct/Visiting) Hunan Normal University and Peking University
[1]New Zealand
[2]China

1. Introduction

Cultural differences are real and arresting. They are noted, discussed and debated in bioethics, as in contemporary social and political life in general. But cultural differences can be very tricky to interpret. Their factual status, moral meanings and political implications are rarely, if ever, as straightforward as they appear. Cultural differences can be seriously misconceived, misinterpreted, misrepresented and misused in various ways. Empirically problematic perceptions, ethically dubious judgments, and practically contentious resolutions can easily become entangled when considering matters of cultural difference. Many works on cross-cultural bioethics have often merely served to reinforce deeply rooted stereotypes and myths regarding both Western and non-Western cultures, especially the latter. A glaring example of such confusion is the appeal to perceived cultural differences as an ethical justification for rejecting those norms perceived as originating in the West and strongly advocated there - such as truth-telling by medical professionals, informed consent, patients' rights, women's rights and human rights in general. It is argued and widely held in certain circles that such practices and values are irrelevant and inapplicable to non-Western societies and cultures.

In this paper, I will critically examine "the cultural differences" argument as it has been formulated against medical truth-telling in the Chinese context. I will demonstrate that, despite its popularity and apparent plausibility, the argument is seriously flawed both descriptively and normatively. Elsewhere, through comparisons between China and the West and supported by extensive primary Chinese materials, I have shown that direct disclosure is far from culturally alien to China and that, on the contrary, there was once a long, though forgotten, tradition of medical truth-telling in China (Nie 2011: Chapter 6). Here, I argue that, even if medical truth-telling were culturally alien to China, as usually assumed, ethical imperatives exist to reform the contemporary mainstream Chinese practice of nondisclosure or indirect disclosure through family members. Moreover, I will offer a Confucian defence of truth-telling as a fundamental ethical principle and a cardinal personal and social virtue which physicians would do well to take seriously. In the process, I expose some common intellectual barriers to cross-cultural understanding: dichotomizing different cultures as "radical others" to one another, promoting the tyranny of existing cultural practices, and obscuring the real ethical issues at stake. To put the matter positively, I seek to present the elements of a more adequate cross-cultural bioethics or a "transcultural bioethics" - an ethics that resists cultural stereotypes, upholds the primacy of morality, and acknowledges the richness, openness and internal heterogeneity of medical ethics in every culture, whether in China or elsewhere.

2. The "cultural differences" argument

It is known far and wide that, in sharp contrast to most Western countries where truthfulness constitutes an essential, even legally required, element of good medical practice, medical professionals in contemporary China (including Hong Kong and Taiwan) customarily withhold from patients crucial information about terminal illnesses such as cancer. Any information given out is usually restricted to family members only, and is often given in an overtly paternalist manner (e.g., Kleinman 1988: 152, Li and Chou 1997, Pang 1998, 1999, Tse, Chong and Fob 2003, Fan and Li 2004, Tang and Lee 2004, Zhu 2005, Zeng, Li, Chen and Fang 2007, Tang et al. 2008).

This situation is not restricted to China. Nondisclosure or indirect disclosure through family members is the mainstream practice in other Asian countries such as Japan and Nepal, as well as in other parts of the world such as the Middle East and Eastern and Southern Europe (e.g. Surbone 1992, Mitsuya 1997, Gongal et al. 2006, Mobereek et al 2008). In different countries or within different ethnic groups within the same country, patients suffering from cancer and other terminal illnesses receive very different levels of information about their diagnosis, prognosis, and therapeutic options (e.g. Macklin 1999, Mitchell 1998, Mystakidou et al. 2004, Tuckett 2004, Hancock et al. 2007, Surbone 2006, 2008). As the title of an editorial by an Italian physician in the journal *Support Care Cancer* characterizes it, there is a "persisting difference in truth telling throughout the world" (Surbone 2004).

According to more recent literature, although "there is a shift in truth-telling attitudes and practice toward greater disclosure of diagnosis to cancer patients worldwide", "partial and nondisclosure is still common in many cultures that are centered on family and community values" (Surbone 2008, 237). Thus this striking cultural difference—direct disclosure in most Western countries vs. non-disclosure or indirect disclosure in most non-Western societies—is still prevalent in the twenty-first century.

It is from acknowledging this cultural divide that the "cultural differences" view, that opposes medical truth-telling in non-Western societies like China, has taken root. Two Chinese medical ethicists put the issue succinctly: "In contrast [with the West], Chinese medical ethics, even today, in theory and in practice, remains committed to hiding the truth as well as to lying when necessary to achieve the family's view of the best interests of the patient" (Fan and Li 2004, 180). Direct truth-telling - the so-called "Western individualistic mode" - is defined as being culturally alien to China and therefore morally unsound because it violates so-called "Chinese familial values".

In Japan, similar arguments have been put forward to reject medical truth-telling and replace it by a family-centered style of informed consent. A major rationale behind the distinction holds that the construal of the self in Japanese and Western culture is to be defined as "interdependent vs. independent" respectively, or, to put it another way, in terms of the family vs. the individual (Akabayashi and Slingsby 2006).

The cultural differences argument against medical truth-telling can take a number of different forms. In the Chinese context, one common argument, in the form of a syllogism, goes like this:

Major premise: Different cultural norms and practices ought to be respected and maintained;

Minor premise: In contrast to the Western practice of direct disclosure regarding terminal illness, the cultural norm in China is nondisclosure or indirect disclosure through family members;

Conclusion: Therefore, medical professionals should refrain from telling Chinese patients the truth about their terminal illness.

A more sophistical version of the argument goes thus:

First premise: Different cultural norms and practices ought to be respected and maintained;

Second premise: Chinese and Western cultures are fundamentally and radically different from each other;

Third premise: Truth-telling is the Western cultural norm and is founded on individualistic Western culture;

Fourth premise: Nondisclosure or indirect disclosure through family members is the Chinese cultural norm and is founded on family-oriented Chinese culture;

Conclusion: Therefore, nondisclosure or indirect disclosure through family members should be maintained and the practice of medical truth-telling rejected in China.

Whatever form it takes, the cultural differences argument consists of two core claims—one descriptive and the other normative. The empirical or *descriptive* claim generalizes secrecy and lying to the sick and dying as the representative and authentic cultural norm for Chinese. The *normative* claim insists the practice of nondisclosure should be maintained in order to respect perceived cultural differences. The descriptive claim is more widely held than the normative one: those who subscribe to the normative claim always found their position on the descriptive claim. Yet, those who accept the descriptive claim do not necessarily agree with the normative claim; they are thus free to take an ethical position against nondisclosure or indirect disclosure.

3. The current debate in China

Defying its contemporary stereotype as a monolithic, changeless nation or (in the famous metaphor of Napoleon) a "sleeping lion", China has always been in a state of flux. In the past three or so decades - a period designated by the Chinese authorities as one of "reform and openness" - the enormous social and economic transformations undergone by China have had a profound impact on the history of both China and the world. On the medical front, the patient-physician relationship, including the handling of medical information relating to incurable and terminal diseases, has undergone a comparable "revolution". In the 1980s when I was a medical student and intern in China, it was standard practice that patients were never told directly about their terminal illness. We were instructed to conceal such a diagnosis and even lie to the sick and dying - for instance, not to write the Chinese character for cancer, *ai,* on the patient's card, but the English abbreviation *Ca*. This cloak of secrecy surrounding the terminally ill was (and still is) referred to by a special quasi-medical term - "protective medical treatment" (*baohuxing yiliao*).

Since the 1990s and especially the early 2000s, however, the practice of withholding crucial medical information has been challenged by patients, medical professionals, and the general public. An historic change is happening in China, a shift from secrecy and lying toward honest and direct disclosure. In 2008, thirteen hospitals throughout China and the premier Chinese journal *Medicine and Philosophy* jointly issued a series of documents on informed consent (*Yixue Yu Zhexu* 2008, 1-12). One of them is entitled "Guiding Principles on Truth-telling to and Consent from Cancer Patients". While it promotes only partial disclosure and insists on the necessity of "appropriate confidentiality" (ibid, 7-8), this document indicates that the Chinese debate on the issue has subtly shifted from *whether* patients should be told about their condition to *when* and *how* they should be best informed.

In many ways, the Chinese debate closely resembles the Western debate of the 1960s and 1970s. As a matter of course, advocates of honest and direct disclosure take up the language of rights - the right of the patient to know and decide. They also call attention to the damage done by secrecy and concealing the truth from patients, as well as the benefits of honest communication for both patients and physicians. On the other side of the debate, defenders of nondisclosure, especially medical professionals and family members, emphasize the duty to protect patients and, at least, to avoid doing harm. It is assumed that the communication of complex and negative medical information is bad for patients' morale, if not beyond their intelligence. It has often been asserted, not only in the mass media but also in the medical and academic literature, that telling the truth about terminal illness frightens and depresses patients, deprives them of hope, and may even shorten their lives. It has been circulated that young women are more vulnerable than other groups and are more likely to commit suicide after learning of a negative prognosis.

The Chinese debate differs in one salient area from that conducted in the West several decades ago: the issue of cultural differences. A common argument invoked to oppose medical truth-telling in China lies in the appeal to cultural differences, in particular to Chinese values and cultural context. Indeed, the invoking of the cultural argument raises a number of questions regarding the current Chinese trend to honest and open disclosure. Is this new development merely an aping of the contemporary Western norm? Is it a consequence of Western cultural hegemony or even of bioethical imperialism? More fundamentally, is this current shift in attitudes merely a change of fashion or is it based on sound moral foundations? If the cultural differences argument against medical truth-telling in China is valid, then current efforts to reform the still widespread practice of secrecy and lying to the sick and dying are heading in the wrong direction.

But the argument against this reform is seriously flawed. In what follows, I reveal and discuss a number of empirical and normative problems with this argument, however appealing it may be on the surface.

4. Dicthotomizing east and west

The cultural differences argument is anchored in and perpetuates a deeply rooted and still prevalent habit of thought: the dichotomizing of the West and the non-West as "radical others" to one another (for a critical examination of what can be called the "fallacy of dichotomizing cultures," see Nie 2011, especially Chapters 1 and 2). In bioethics, this polarization of East and West is manifested in the popular but specious idea of "Western individualist bioethics" vs. "Asian communitarian bioethics" (Nie 2007). According to this way of thinking, the dominant practice or official position of a given culture or social group is deemed the authentic representative of the culture or social group concerned. And the differences between and among cultures are perceived to be radical, fundamental, and largely incompatible with each other. As a result, the actual richness and great internal plurality of a given culture and the complexity of cultural differences within and between different groups are oversimplified and all too often seriously distorted.

Drawing on and perpetuating this cultural dichotomy, the cultural differences argument against medical truth-telling in the Chinese context has crudely distorted the historical and socio-cultural realities of both China and the West. As the first part of my comparative study of medical truth-telling has uncovered (Nie 2011, Chapter 6), historically speaking, it is simply incorrect to claim that truth-telling is the representative Western cultural norm while it is culturally alien to China. Far from being an age-old cultural tradition, in the West medical truth-telling did not become the accepted standard until the 1970s or even later - it has a history of a few decades only. And, on the other side, totally contrary to what has been universally assumed and presented both inside and outside China, the traditional practice and norm of Chinese culture and medical ethics was for physicians to disclose their diagnosis and prognosis of terminal illness truthfully and directly to patients. A great deal of primary historical material, including the biographies of ancient medical sages and hundreds of celebrated physicians in different dynasties (Chen 1991[1723]), reveals a well-established Chinese tradition of medical truth-telling that dates back at least twenty-six centuries. Ironically, the contemporary mainstream Chinese practice of nondisclosure as a "historical" phenomenon has a great deal to do with an older Western norm of concealing medical information.

5. Chinese patients want to know the truth

Sociologically, the cultural differences view has assumed that Chinese patients are not only kept in ignorance of their condition, but even prefer things this way. However, in total contrast to this assumption, the great majority of Chinese people, like Westerners, want to know the truth about their medical condition if suffering from serious illness.

In a telephone survey of 2674 Chinese households conducted in Hong Kong in 1995, 95% of 1138 interviewees aged between 18 and 65 indicated that they would prefer knowing their medical diagnosis, even if the outlook was grave. The same proportion said they would object if their family only was informed, while they themselves were not told. And 97% of respondents would want to know their prognosis. The researchers concluded that the patterns of preference shown by Chinese people in Hong Kong were "very similar to those reported in studies on Western populations" (Fielding and Hung 1996). Taiwanese cancer patients also expressed a strong preference for medical professionals to tell them the truth, even before informing relatives (Tang and Lee 2004).

The same is true of mainland Chinese. In the early 2000s, speaking to a class of about 60 students, mostly postgraduates, in one of the leading ethics programs in China (in Hunan Normal University located in Changsha, a central southern Chinese city), I asked if they would like to know the truth if they were diagnosed with a terminal illness. A large majority responded "yes" (about 50), and only a handful said "no".

Despite some deficiencies in sample selections and research design, many extensive surveys conducted throughout mainland China clearly indicate the preference of the great (or even overwhelming) majority of Chinese patients suffering from terminal illness to be fully apprised of the medical facts about their condition. A survey of 311 cancer patients in Guangzhou in southeast China found that 72.99% believed that patients should be fully informed; 24.12% responded that the decision should depend on the wishes of the patients themselves; and only 2.89% thought that patients should not be told about their cancer diagnosis (Huang, Wang, Zhang, Lü and Li 2001). In a survey conducted in Shenyang, northeast China, involving 198 hospitalized elderly cancer patients and 312 family members, 94% of patients and 82.7% of family members considered it essential for the truth to be told about their terminal illness, and 97% of patients and 90.4% of family members believed that the sharing of accurate medical information would improve the outcomes of treatment (Gao, Zou and Yang 2006). Another survey of 302 cancer patients in Wuhan, central South China, concluded that, in general, cancer patients are very keen to know the truth about their illness and that the practice of "protective treatment" had resulted in distrust of medical professionals and increased concerns about the seriousness of their condition (Zeng, Zhou, Hong, Xiang, and Fang 2008).

However, the cultural difference view is accurate on one point - in China, most medical professionals and the majority of family members are unwilling to inform patients truthfully (see the survey results presented below). Interestingly, when they were asked whether or not they would like to know the truth if they were themselves had been diagnosed with terminal illness, the great majority said they would want to know. A survey conducted in 2004 among 180 nurses in Shandong in Northeast coastal China showed that, when imagining themselves as patients, they would prefer to be informed even though, *as medical professionals*, they would hesitate to tell the truth to their own patients (Zhu 2005, 73). When the nurses put themselves in their patients' shoes, the overwhelming majority of them, 92.6%, preferred to know the diagnosis and prognosis of severe and terminal illness. However, when asked whether they *as nurses* should inform their patients about *their* adverse medical conditions, 71.6% said that they would withhold the truth. When asked to imagine themselves as patients' family members, only 2.5% would speak directly and immediately, 69.1% would choose to tell the truth after prevaricating for a time, and 28.4% would not disclose the condition in any circumstances (Ibid). A survey of 634 doctors and nurses, conducted in Wuhan, again illustrates that medical professionals are reluctant to speak candidly about cancer; that patients are aware of that they have insufficient knowledge about their medical condition; and that physicians are inclined to let family members, rather than patients, make important decisions (Zeng, Li, Chen, and Fang 2007).

As presented in the second section of this chapter, there are signs that the attitudes of mainland Chinese medical professionals are changing. In 2009, lecturing to a class of 50 medical students at Peking University Health Science Centre, a leading medical school in China located in Beijing, I asked the class whether they would tell patients about their diagnosis and prognosis of terminal illness. The great majority answered "yes" by raising their hands.

Other surveys confirm the disparity between patients' wishes on the one hand and the reluctance of family members on the other. In a survey of 175 patients and 238 family members visiting a hospital clinic in Beijing (He, Wang, Tian, Zhou and Wang 2009), 42% of patients wanted to be told immediately after a diagnosis of cancer was confirmed, 31.4% wanted both patients and family members to be told together, and 26.3% preferred that only family members be informed. However, only 2.1% of family members wanted the diagnosis to be communicated directly to the patient - although 16.4% wanted both patients and family members to be told. The contrasts in this survey are stark: whereas nearly three quarters of patients wanted to be informed, either alone or with family members, more than three quarters of family members preferred that doctors inform them alone. In another survey of 194 family members of recently diagnosed and hospitalized cancer patients, 57.7% disagreed and 42.3% agreed that patients should be told (Sun, Li, Sun and Chang 2007). A further survey of 382 patients and 482 relatives in Chengdu, Southwestern China, indicates that cancer patients were more likely than family members to believe that patients should be informed (early stage, 90.8% vs 69.9%; terminal stage, 60.5% vs 34.4%) and that most participants preferred being told immediately after the diagnosis (Jiang, Li and Li et al. 2007).

One ethical question that arises from the disagreement between patients, their families, and health care providers, disclosed by these studies is - what should be done when patients want to know about their condition but medical professionals and relatives prefer to withhold information and even lie to them? In Chinese culture, the Golden Rule taught by Confucius is widely known and respected: "Do not impose on others what you do not wish for yourself" (*jishuo buyu, wushi yuren*). If the general preference of Chinese people for knowing the truth about terminal illness is interpreted as a wish not be lied to or to remain in ignorance, then, according to the Golden Rule, it is ethically unacceptable for medical professionals and relatives to impose on patients what they consider to be in the patients' best interests, regardless of what patients themselves prefer.

Another ethical question arises over the significant proportion of patients who prefer *not* to know about their prognosis. The short answer is that one should not impose the unpalatable truth upon this group. To ignore the wish not to know is as wrong as dismissing the desire to know. Perhaps pre-diagnosis informed consent is required to address this.

6. Harms done by secrecy and untruthfulness

As Tolstoy's *The Death of Ivan Ilyich* and Solzhenitsyn's *Cancer Ward* so vividly illustrate, patients can often sense the seriousness of their illness even though both medical professionals and relatives strive to keep the truth from them. My own experience as an intern at a Chinese county hospital in the 1980s confirms the reality of this instinctive awareness of their condition by patients. In fact, a major practical difficulty of hiding the truth in these circumstances is that it is almost impossible to carry out successfully. Humans communicate with each other not only through language, but also through their social context, body language, and by many other means. The specialised wards and hospitals that patients find themselves in, and the gestures of medical professionals, relatives and friends can easily reveal the truth, despite all efforts to hide it. For the patients concerned, whatever others may tell them, the secrecy surrounding their treatment reveals a truth of paramount importance - their illness is serious.

Even if it were feasible to hide the truth from patients, the practice of nondisclosure—the norm in China today—should be reversed because it is harmful to patients. On the one hand, the advocates of nondisclosure have offered no compelling evidence of its benefits for patients or their families. On the other hand, they often downplay or ignore the enormous harm that the practice of nondisclosure and evasion has caused to patients, families, the medical profession, and society at large. In addition to dismissing patients' wish to know, the practice of nondisclosure increases the feelings of abandonment of those suffering from terminal illness and undermines the bonds of social trust, in particular those between patients and medical professionals.

For the cultural differences argument, the ethical rationale for disclosure turns on the question of individual rights and personal autonomy. The norm of medical truth-telling is thus arguably not applicable to those societies and cultures where the language of individual rights and autonomy is largely absent. It is true that, politically, the shift from nondisclosure to disclosure that occurred in most Western countries around the 1970s had a great deal to do with the patients' rights movement. And, in bioethics, disclosure and informed consent are often theoretically justified out of respect for the patient's autonomy, a leading principle in the discipline. However, it is a mistake to regard the ethical rationale for direct disclosure as wholly based on the notions of individual rights and autonomy. There are other sound ethical reasons for direct disclosure—for instance, the principle of beneficence, a fundamental value for almost every healing system and medical ethics tradition worldwide.

Although often overlooked in cross-cultural discussions of truth-telling and informed consent, a major factor in the historical shift toward disclosure in the West was the practical necessity for effective (but not overly aggressive) therapeutic intervention. Jay Katz's *The Silent World of Doctor and Patient*, a classic of bioethics, has highlighted this crucial point. The practice of truth-telling and informed consent is grounded not only in the principle of autonomy or self-determination, but also in good therapeutic management in face of the problem of uncertainty in medicine and the new challenges that have arisen in caring for seriously ill and dying patients. Nondisclosure and untruthfulness are not ethically justifiable because "[t]he iatrogenic deprivation of information makes a powerful contribution to patients' sense of abandonment." (Ibid, 212)

Doctors' ready retreat behind silence—apparent to patients by doctors' demeanor when they keep most of their thoughts to themselves, deprive patients of vital information, or pat patients on the back and assure them that everything will be all right and they need not worry—makes patients feel disregarded, ignored, patronized, and dismissed. (Ibid, 209-210)

In the words of two other authors, "Tacitly to impose silence, denial, deception, and isolation upon the dying patient may itself cause suffering and bring about bereavement of the dying, a state of premortem loneliness, emotional abandonment, and withdrawn interest" (cited in Katz 2002: 222). The practice of nondisclosure thus serves medical professionals' interests more than those of patients. Disclosure and informed consent, on the other hand, "seek to protect patients from the ravages and pain of abandonment" (Ibid, 208).

In the late nineteenth century, Tolstoy imaginatively rendered the detrimental effects of lying to the patient with terminal illness:

> Ivan Ilyich suffered most of all from the lie, the lie, for some reason, everyone accepted, that he was not dying but was simply ill, and that if he stayed calm and underwent treatment he could expect good results. Yet he knew that regardless of what was done, all he could expect was more agonizing suffering and death. And he was tortured by this lie, tortured by the fact that they refused to acknowledge what he and everyone else knew, that they wanted to lie about his horrible condition and to force him to become a part of that lie. This lie, a lie perpetrated on the eve of his death, a lie that was bound to degrade the awesome, solemn act of his dying to the level of their social calls, their draperies, and the sturgeon they ate for dinner, was an excruciating torture for Ivan Ilyich. And, oddly enough, many times when they were going through their acts with him he came within a hairbreadth of shouting: "Stop your lying! You and I know that I'm dying, so at least stop lying!" (Tolstoy 1981, 102-103)

Acknowledging to patients the seriousness of their medical condition may not be caring or healing in itself (although one could argue that it is), but it is at least the starting point for any good caring and healing regime. Medical professionals and other caregivers may lack the power to truly relieve the suffering of gravely ill and dying patients, but, as Ivan Ilyich urged, they can "at least stop lying".

Those who defend the practice of nondisclosure in China may contest that Chinese patients do not feel the abandonment, loneliness and agony that Ivan Ilyich or Western patients experienced when deprived of critical medical information. But, unless convincing empirical evidence is provided for this imagined cultural difference, one must assume that Chinese patients do not differ radically from their counterparts in the West in this regard.

The major concern in contemporary China, as in the West a few decades ago, is that open and direct disclosure may harm patients. Yet, in Western countries where medical truth-telling has now become firmly established it has been shown that concerns over the presumed psychological and physical harms to patients are in most cases unfounded. And it need hardly be said that such paternalistic attitudes seriously underestimate the intelligence, resilience and resolve of patients suffering from terminal illness in dealing with the realities of death and dying.

Lying has a further serious detrimental effect - the harm done to the patient-physician relationship. Social trust is the foundation of any good communal life. Lying to patients undermines their trust in medical professionals, just as lying in public life does lethal damage to the sustaining and nourishing of social trust. So nondisclosure and untruthfulness can hardly be justified by either "individualistic" or "communitarian" values.

7. The question of family

As we have seen, a key element of the cultural difference view that defends the Chinese practice of nondisclosure stems from a highly legitimate and important concern - the interests and integrity of the family. However, a number of the assumptions and assertions involved in defending this concern are empirically problematic and ethically misleading. Although detailed discussion of the role of the family in relation to bioethics from a Chinese-Western comparative perspective needs much more space, I wish to at least raise a few questions on the subject here.

Firstly, based on the popular dichotomy of China and the West as "radical others", the cultural differences argument posits a cross-cultural distinction, asserting that the family is central or even unique in Chinese culture but not so in the West. Those who would make this assertion are very selective and arbitrary in their choice ofcultural traditions within China and the West. Several major Chinese schools of thought and socio-political movements such as Daoism, Moism, the New Culture Movement in the early twentieth century and Chinese socialism - both in its ideology and in its political-economic system - have all challenged the primacy of the family. At the same time, the essential role of the family in Western civilization (e.g., in Judeo-Christian tradition) as well as in Western bioethics has very often been downplayed and even dismissed. The truth is that, both as an essential social institution and as a cardinal moral value, the family has always been a vital element of any society or culture, whether in the East or in the West.

Secondly, the practice of nondisclosure in China has been attributed to the value placed by Confucianism on the primacy of the family. Yet, as I showed elsewhere (Nie 2011), the well-established Chinese tradition of open and direct disclosure on medical matters was endorsed by one of the key Confucian moral ideals, that of *cheng* (truthfulness, sincerity).

Thirdly and most importantly, the argument about the family assumes that the practice of nondisclosure or indirect disclosure is more beneficial to the family than that of direct disclosure. However, there is no empirical evidence to support this. Secrecy and lying can be very harmful to family relationships as vividly portrayed, once again, in Tolstoy's *Death of Ivan Illich*. On the contrary, a strong case can be made that direct disclosure may better serve families affected, and family values, in than nondisclosure and deceit.

Drawing on the classic work of Sissela Bok (1989 [1978]), who condemns deception in public life, including lying to dying patients, as both ethically unjustifiable and practically harmful, some Western scholars have challenged the "cultural difference" view of truth-telling to the sick and dying in the Chinese context (e.g. Wear 2007). Still, we are warned to "studiously avoid presuming to take a firm stand" on lobbying for truth-telling as a general rule in Chinese society because the available data allegedly do not give a clear picture on two crucial points at the heart of the realted ethical dilemma: what Chinese patients typically want, and whether medical truth-telling will undermine the traditional Chinese family (Ibid).

However, as discussed above, we do have reliable data on the preference of the majority of Chinese to know the truth about terminal illness. As for the relationship between truth-telling and the family, the practice of direct disclosure in the West over the past several decades suggests that disclosure in itself does not necessarily harm the family as a social institution or as a locus of moral value. Truth-telling can empower family members to better support dying patients, attend to the needs and wellbeing of their loved ones, and diminish the feelings of abandonment and loneliness experienced by their suffering relative. In such difficult times when, as a Chinese saying expresses it, the whole family suffers if a single member is in pain (*yiren xiangyu, mandang bule*), truth-telling can strengthen, rather than weaken, the bonds of love and interdependence among family members.

8. The Confucian morality of truthfulness and its ethical implication for medical practice

The contemporary Chinese practice of non-disclosure or indirect disclosure has been presented and argued to be justifiable and preferable according to Confucianism (e.g. Fan and Li 2004). However, this interpretation of Confucianism is historically groundless (see Nie 2011: Chapter 6) and normatively wrong and misleading. In other words, the contemporary dominant - though challenged - practice in China cannot be justified by the ethical principles and ideals of major Chinese moral, political and spiritual traditions such as Confucianism.

In Confucianism, the highest moral ideals or principles are *ren* (humanity, humaneness), *yi* (righteousness) and *li* (the correct performance of rites), although scholars disagree about which has primacy (for a discussion of Confucian professional ethics of medicine, see Nie 2011: Chapters 11 and 12). While *chengxin* (truthfulness, honesty, trustworthiness or sincerity), another virtue highly regarded in Confucianism, is often used as a single phrase in modern Chinese, in classical Chinese *cheng* and *xin* are two closely related but different concepts, especially in Confucian tradition. Confucius himself discussed *xin* frequently in the *Analects*. While it rarely appears in the *Analects*, *cheng* is a key term in Neo-Confucianism and in other two Confucian classics, *The Great Learning* and *The Doctrine of the Means*.

The necessity of acquiring *xin* is a major theme in the *Analects*. According to a contemporary Chinese scholar, the term - meaning honesty, faithfulness and truthfulness - appears at least 24 times in the "Bible of China" (Yang1980, 257). The other fundamental Confucian concepts of *ren*, *li* and *yi* appear 108, 74, and 24 times in the *Analects* respectively (Ibid, 221, 311, 291). Since the early Han Dynasty (c. the 2nd century BCE) when Confucianism was established as the official ideology of the state, *xin* has been regarded as the fifth of the Five Cardinal Virtues (*wuchang*) of Confucianism. Confucius used the metaphor of the yoke or horse harness to illustrate the importance of honesty and truthfulness for both individuals and social life (II, 23):

The Master said, "I do not know how a man without truthfulness is to get on. How can a large carriage be made to go without the cross-bar for yoking the oxen to, or a small carriage without the arrangement for yoking the horses?" (Legge 1971 [1893], 153)

Confucius placed a very high value on *xin*, stating that "No human being can stand without truthfulness" (XII, 7) and, in *The Great Learning* (III, 3), "In communication with people, he [ie, the truthful person] abides in faithfulness."

While the term *cheng* (sincerity, authenticity or truthfulness) is rarely mentioned in the *Analects*, it is a crucial concept in other Confucian classics and for Confucianism in general. The term embodies a complex nexus of metaphysical, ethical, psychological, and spiritual meanings, as the following quote from *The Doctrine of the Mean* (XX, 18) indicates:

Sincerity [truthfulness] is the way of Heaven. The attainment of sincerity is the way of men. He who possesses sincerity, is he who, without an effort, hits what is right, and apprehends, without the exercise of thought; - he is the sage who naturally and easily embodies the *right* way. He who attains to sincerity, is he who chooses what is good, and firmly holds it fast. (Legge 1971[1893], 413; emphasis original)

Philosophically, this passage is comparable to Kant's discussion of "the good will". Still, however sophisticated the ramifications of the term may be, at the most basic level, like *xin*, *cheng* equates to one of the most fundamental moral maxims endorsed by most if not all human societies and ethical systems: be honest and, at the very least, do not deceive.

It is important to point out that, while the ethical principle of truthfulness is essential for Confucianism, this value is not absolute. In certain situations, concealing the truth is certainly an acceptable course, even a praiseworthy one. According to a story in the *Analects* (XIII, 18):

The duke of Sheh [Ye], informed Confucius, saying, "Among us here there are those who may be styled upright [or just] in their conduct. If their father has stolen a sheep, they will bear witness to the fact."

Confucius said, "Among us, in our part of the country, those who are upright are different from this. The father conceals the misconduct of the son, and the son conceals the misconduct of the father. Uprightness [or justice] is to be found in this." (Legge 1971 [1893], 270).

In one of the early dialogues of Plato, *Euthyphro*, Socrates challenged a similar belief that it is right to indict one's father for committing manslaughter. Many commentators, ancient, modern and contemporary, have debated the rationale behind the position taken by Confucius here. For the purposes of our discussion, the point is that, in striking contrast to Kant's deontological ethics, truthfulness is not an absolute value in Confucianism.

What are the implications of the Confucian morality of truthfulness for medical practice regarding whether medical professionals should tell the patients the dire diagnosis and prognosis? First and foremost, as a general maxim for medical practice, healthcare professionals should abide by truthfulness as strictly as they can, following the consensus established by traditional Chinese medical ethics over the centuries. To deceive patients for motives of personal gain is always absolutely wrong and morally corrupt. Even when delivering painful news, as in the diagnosis and prognosis of terminal illness, truthfulness should not be easily set aside and medical practitioners should practice open and direct disclosure as a general rule, following the norm of the ancient Chinese medical sages.

Moreover, following the example of the systematic modern Chinese text on the professional ethics of medicine (Nie 2011: Chapter 6), a careful distinction should be made between lying (or deception) and concealing the truth. Ethically, there is a subtle but significant difference between these two; in the words of a Chinese idiom, "an error the breadth of a single hair can lead someone astray by a thousand miles".

The principle of truthfulness should be breached only in exceptional circumstances, such as when complete candour would lead to serious danger for the patient, such as confirmed risk of suicide due to breaking bad news. For Confucian medical ethics the highest ideal is *ren*, as articulated in the ethical definition of healing: "medicine as the art of humanity or humaneness". Nevertheless, the burden of proof should fall on those who believe that the principle of open and direct disclosure should be breached in order to avoid perceived risks to the patient. I have presented overwhelming evidence in this chapter that the great majority of Chinese patients want information about their medical condition. And we have seen that a conspiracy of silence or outright deception by family members and medical professionals can do great harm to patients. So those cases in which the truth needs to be concealed are likely to be rare. Cases where patients need to be deceived should be even rarer.

Yet, while most Chinese patients would prefer to know the truth about their medical condition, there is still a significant proportion of patients who prefer to be kept in ignorance about their prognosis. This raises a moral question as well as a medical challenge. As mentioned in Section 5, the short answer is that one should not impose the unpalatable truth upon this group; and to ignore a patient's wish not to know is as wrong as dismissing their legitimate desire to know. From a cross-cultural perspective, patients who subscribe to the "ignorance is bliss" mentality can be found not only in China but also in the West. On this point, it is also worth pointing out that, as far as Confucianism is concerned, the concept of *cheng* includes a criticism and even a condemnation of self-deception.

The radical level of disagreement revealed in the hospital survey results cited above provides evidence of a genuine moral dilemma for contemporary Chinese: that is, as discussed at the end of Section 5, what should be done when patients want to know the truth about their condition but medical professionals and relatives prefer to withhold information and even lie to them? According to the Golden Rule in Confucianism, "Do not impose on others what you do not wish for yourself," medical professionals should not obstruct the wish of patients in order to achieve what they believe to be in the best interest of patients.

Placing the onus of disclosure on family members in cases of terminal illness, a practice that is widespread in China and favourably endorsed by the advocates of the cultural differences argument, raises additional ethical questions. For instance, is this really in the patient's best interests, or for the convenience of medical professionals? Telling patients the truth about their serious condition is an art; however caring and experienced he or she may be, no physician will be perfect at this. As the 1847 Code of Ethics of the American Medical Association recommends, it is not ethically sound for physicians to delegate this difficult task wholly to family members. Apart from their obvious lack of systematic training in medicine and counselling, most importantly, lay relatives may lack the necessary professional and personal distance often critical for imparting sensitive information in an empathic way. Chinese medical professionals need to change their practice on this. Shunning a professional duty merely because of its difficulty is unacceptable, ethically and professionally. If the real motivation for "familist" practice is simply the convenience of medical professionals, then the practice clearly needs reform. For Chinese medical practitioners, the basic requirement of the Confucian medical ideal, "medicine as the art of humanity", is to fulfil their professional duties, however challenging they may be.

9. The tyranny of culture vs. the primacy of morality

Respecting perceived cultural differences constitutes a major ethical stumbling block to implementing the practice of direct and truthful medical disclosure in non-Western societies (and non-European groups within Western countries). By this logic, the current mainstream cultural practice is proffered as a sufficient ethical rationale to reject medical truth-telling. In other words, the "cultural difference" proponents attempt to bypass the moral difficulties involved by substituting statements about cultural practices for serious ethical examination. In this age of Western cultural hegemony, it is extremely important to respect different cultural practices, especially non-Western ones. However, an ethical dilemma arises when cultural practices conflict with moral imperatives. The cultural difference argument privileges cultural practices over ethical mandates; it implies, if not holds, that whatever is culturally authentic is automatically ethically defensible. This tyranny of culture over ethics can easily lead to moral relativism and even ethical nihilism. According to the logic of the cultural difference view, slavery in human history; gender discrimination and many other forms of discrimination, which are found in almost all human societies; the West's colonization of the non-Western world; the Third Reich in Germany; and foot-binding in Chinese history - to list just a few examples - are all ethically justifiable because all these practices were or still are culturally genuine and even unique.

More crucially, respecting cultural norms and practices can actually work against the fundamental values of a given culture and society. For both Confucianism and Daoism, the two major indigenous Chinese moral and political traditions, it is not existing cultural practices that should be privileged, but whatever is morally right. For Confucianism and Daoism, the most fundamental value is precisely the primacy of ethics and morality over existing social and cultural practices, rather than the other way around. The moral imperative of the Dao (Tao, literally "the Way") or the *Tianming* (the mandate of Heaven) is superior to the claims of any cultural and social practices, whether Western or Eastern. The basic task and highest calling of ethics is, first of all, to identify which socio-cultural practices are morally justifiable and which are not.

10. Conclusion

Taking a universalist ethical position on human rights and patients' rights, other bioethicists have forcefully argued the importance of truth-telling and informed consent internationally, in China as well (Macklin 1999). This may be seen as a kind of outside perspective. In this paper, my stance is from the inside out.

My aim is not to dispute the existence of widely acknowledged cultural differences in China and the West regarding medical truth-telling. Rather, the key question for me is *how this prima facie cultural difference – direct disclosure vs. non-disclosure or indirect disclosure – should be interpreted historically, sociologically and ethically.* In particular, I have demonstrated that, despite its popularity and apparent plausibility, the cultural differences argument against medical truth-telling in China is seriously flawed at both the descriptive and normative levels. It has oversimplified and distorted both the historical and socio-cultural realities, including the role of family, in both China and the West. It has mis-presented and mis-interpreted the standpoints of such major Chinese traditions as Confucianism on the subject. Historically, it has ignored the venerable Chinese tradition of direct truth-telling and, sociologically, it has dismissed the wishes of the great majority of Chinese patients who want to know the truth about their prospects. Ethically, it has obscured critical moral problems involved in nondisclosure and deception by medical professionals, and it promotes the tyranny of existing socio-cultural practices over ethics and acceptable morality.

Therefore, the contemporary Chinese practice of concealing the truth and even lying to patients about their terminal illness, no matter how widespread, ought to be critically examined, vigorously challenged, and systematically reformed. Culturally, the shift toward honest and direct disclosure now occurring in China is not so much -or at least not just- following a Western pathway, but constitutes a return to a neglected indigenous tradition (for a detailed discussion of this forgotten Chinese tradition, see Nie 2011, Chapter 6). More importantly, even if it were proven to be culturally alien to China as universally assumed, the norm of truth-telling should be instituted on the basis of the ethical imperatives presented in this paper.

As for cross-cultural bioethics, if I have appeared to argue that all cultures are fundamentally the same and that cultural differences do not matter, I would like to say that this is not my intention. My point is that Chinese and Western cultures *are* different, but not in the ways suggested by popular stereotypes, not in the sense of their being "radical others" to one another. As this study of medical truth-telling in China and other research projects have illustrated, Chinese-Western cultural differences are far more complicated, subtle, intriguing - and thus more difficult to grasp and articulate - than facile overgeneralizations. Rather than being homogenous and static, Chinese culture, like any other human culture, has always been internally heterogeneous, full of contradictory elements, changing over time, influenced by and borrowing elements from foreign cultures, open to new possibilities, and subject to ethical scrutiny and developing moral ideals. The complexity of cultural differences as indicated in medical truth-telling in China in comparison with the West calls for a more adequate cross-cultural bioethics or a "transcultural bioethics": an ethics that resists cultural stereotypes, cherishes the common humanity, upholds the primacy of morality, and acknowledges the richness, internal diversity, dynamism and openness of medical ethics in every culture, whether in China, the West or elsewhere (for these general points, see Nie 2005, 2007, 2009, and especially 2011).

11. A Personal note

I would like to end this paper on a personal note. In the late 1980s, the father of a former medical school classmate and good friend of mine was suffering the final stages of lung cancer. A psychiatrist himself, without any knowledge of the new practice of disclosure in the West, my friend informed his father of the diagnosis and prognosis - something his father's doctors and nurses never did. In taking this step, my friend set out bravely in defiance of the dominant social and medical norm of nondisclosure, and unknowingly travelled a way that ancient Chinese medical sages had walked more than twenty centuries ago. At the time, I should have questioned him further about his courageous decision to choose this unorthodox route. But our discussions were kept brief - after all, it is never easy to talk about the death of a loved one. Now it has become impossible for me to continue the dialogue. Having just celebrated his 31th birthday, and when working as a visiting physician in Japan in 1994, my friend was hit by a car while riding a bicycle and died from his injuries.

This paper is humbly dedicated to Dr Zou Xinxin (1963-1994), a brilliant physician and friend. If only I could have had the benefit of his endorsement and criticism.

12. Acknowledgements

The expanded version of this chapter will be included in my forthcoming book, *Medical Ethics in China: A Transcultural Interpretation*, to be published by Routledge. This work is a part of a larger research project on medical ethics in China, financially supported by a University of Otago Research Grant. I am very grateful to Li Hongwen in Beijing for his research assistance in search of Chinese materials and Dr Paul Sorrell in Dunedin for his professional editing. Parts of materials have been presented as invited speeches at the 7th Beijing Forum, at a symposium organized by Giuliana Fuscaldo, Lynn Gillam and Sarah Russell for the 10th World Congress of Bioethics, and at the second seminar of the New Zealand Ministry of Health Pacific Health Leadership. I gratefully acknowledge the organizers and the audiences of these events for their interest in my work and for their helpful questions and comments.

13. References

Akabayashi A. and B.T. Slingsby. (2006). Informed Consent Revisited: Japan and the U.S. *American Journal of Bioethics,* Vol. 6, No. 1(Jan-Feb 2006), pp.9-14, ISSN 1526-5161, eISSN 1536-0075.

Bok. S. (1978). *Lying: Moral Choice in Public and Private Life.* New York: Vintage Books. ISBN-10: 0375705287, ISBN-13: 978-0375705281

Chen, Menglei. (1991). [1723]. *Gujin Tushu Jicheng Yibu Quanlu* (A Collection of Ancient and Modern Books, Section on Medicine), Book 12: General Discussions (Volumes 501-520 in original), Beijing: People's Health Press. (In Chinese)

Fan, R. and B. Li. (2004). Truth Telling in Medicine: The Confucian View. *Journal of Medicine and Philosophy,* Vol. 29, No.2, (April 2004), pp. 179-193, ISSN 0360-5310, eISSN 1744-5019.

Fielding, R. and J. Hung. (1996). Preference for Information and Involvement in Decisions during Cancer Care among a Hong Kong Chinese Population. *Psycho-, Oncology* Vol. 5, No.4, (December 1996), pp. 321-329, ISSN: 1057-9249, eISSN 1099- 1611.

Gao, B., D. Zou, and L. Yang. (2006). A Study of Methods and Timing with Regard to Informing Elderly Cancer Patients. *Nursing Journal of Chinese People's Liberation Army.* No. 10. (in Chinese)

Gongal, R. P. Vaidya, R. Jha, O. Raijbhandary & M. Watson. (2006).Informing patients about cancer in Nepal: what do people prefer. *Palliative Medicine,* Vol.20, No.4, (June 2006), pp. 471- 476, ISSN 0269-2163, eISSN 1477-030X.

Hancock, K. et al. (2007). Truth-telling in discussing prognosis in advanced life- limiting illness: a systematic review. *Palliative Medicine,* Vol. 21, No.6, (September 2007), pp. 507-517, ISSN 0269-2163, eISSN 1477-030X.

He, R., Y. Wang, Y. Tian, C. Zhou, H. Wang. (2009). The Preferences of Chinese Patients and their Relatives Regarding the Disclosure of Cancer Diagnoses. *Chinese Journal of Clinical Oncology and Rehabilitation.* No. 3. (in Chinese)

Hern, H.E. Jr., B.A. Koenig, L.J. Moore, & P.A. Marshall. (1998). The Difference That Culture Can Make in End-of-Life Decision Making. *Cambridge Quarterly of Healthcare Ethics* Vol. 7, No.1,(Winter 1998), pp. 27-40, ISSN 0963-1801, eISSN 1469-2147.

Huang, X., X. Wang, Y. Zhang, B. Lü, and T. Li. (2001). Information Needs of Cancer Patients: Whether and How to Disclosure the Diagnosis of Cancer. *Chinese Journal of Mental Health* No. 4. (in Chinese)

Jiang, Y., C. Liu, J-Y Li, et al. (2007). Different attitudes of Chinese patients and their families toward truth telling of different stage of cancer. *Psycho-Oncology,* Vol. 16, No. 10, (October 2007), pp. 928-936, ISSN: 1057-9249, eISSN 1099-1611.

Jotkowitz, A., S. Click and B. Gezundheit. (2006). Truth-telling in a Culturally Divers World. *Cancer Investigation* 24:786-789.

Kagaw-Singer, M. and L.J. Blackhall. (2001). Negotiating Cross-Cultural Issues at the End of Life: "You Got to Go Where He Lives". *Journal of American Medical Association,*Vol. 286, No.23, (December 2001), pp. 2993-3001, ISSN 0098-7484, eISSN 1538-3598.

Katz, J. (2002) (first edition 1984). *The Silent World of Doctor and Patient* (with a new foreword by A. M. Capron). Baltimore and London: Johns Hopkins University Press. ISBN 978- 4020-8603-8, eISBN 978-4020-8604-5, Springer.

Kleinman, A. 1988. *The Illness Narratives.* New York: Basic Books. ISBN 0-465-03202-8, ISBN 0-465-03204-4. United States of America.

Legge, J. (tran) (1971) [1893], *The Confucian Analects, The Great Learning and The Doctrine of the Mean,* New York: Dove.

Li, S., and J-L Chou. (1997). Communication with the Cancer Patient in China. *Annals of New York Academy of Sciences,* Vol. 809,(February 1997), pp. 243-248 ISSN 0077-8923, eISSN 1749-6632.

Macklin, R. (1999). *Against Relativism: Cultural Diversity and the Search for Ethical Universals in Medicine.* New York and Oxford: Oxford University Press, ISBN 0-19-511632-J, NY.

Mitchell. J. (1998). Cross-cultural Issues in the Disclosure of Cancer. *Cancer Practice* 6(3): 153-160.

Moberireek A.F. et al. (2008). Information disclosure and decision-making: the Middle East versus the Far East and the West. *Journal of Medical Ethics* Vol.34, No.4, (April 2008), pp. 225-229, ISSN 0306-6800, eISSN 1473-4257.

Mystakidou, K., E. Parpa, E. Tsilika, E. Katsouda, and L. Vlahos. (2004). Cancer information disclosure in different culture context. *Support Care Cancer,* Vol. 12, No.3, (March 2004), pp. 147-154, ISSN 0941-4355, eISSN 1433-7339.

Nie, JB. (2011) (forthcoming). Medical Ethics in China: A Transcultural Interpretation. London and New York: Routledge.

Nie, JB. (2009). The Discourses of Practitioners in China. in Robert Baker and Larry McCullough, eds., *The Cambridge World History of Medical Ethics*, New York and London: Cambridge University Press. Chapter 21, pp. 335-344.

Nie, JB. (2007). The Specious Idea of an Asian Bioethics: Beyond Dichotomizing East and West, in R.E. Ashcroft, A. Dawson, H. Draper and J.R. McMillan, eds. *Principles of Heath Care Ethics,* Second Edition, London: John Wiley & Sons. pp. 143-149.

Nie, JB. (2005). *Behind the Silence: Chinese Voices on Abortion*. Lanham and Oxford: Rowman & Littlefield.

Pang, M.S. (1998). Information Disclosure: The Moral Experience of Nurses in China. *Nursing Ethics,* Vol. 5, No.4, (July 1998), pp.347-361, ISSN 0969-7330, eISSN 1477-0989.

Pang, M.S. (1999). Protective truthfulness: the Chinese way of safeguarding patients in informed treatment decisions. *Journal of Medical Ethics,* Vol.25, No.3, (June 1999), pp. 247-253, ISSN 0306-6800, eISSN 1473-4257.

Surbone, A. (1992). Letter from Italy: Truth Telling to the Patient. *JAMA,* Vol. 268, No.13, (October 1992), pp. 1661-2 ISSN 0098-7484, eISSN 1538-3598.

Surbone. A. (2004). Persisting differences in truth telling throughout the world. *Support Care Cancer,* Vol.12, No.3, (March 2004), pp.143-146. ISSN 0941-4355, eISSN 1433-7339.

Surbone, A. (2006). Telling the Truth to Patients with Cancer: What is the Truth. *Lancet Oncology,* Vol. 7, No. 11 (November 2006), pp. 944-50, ISSN 1470-2045, eISSN 1474-5488.

Surbone, A. (2008). Cultural Aspects of Communication in Cancer Care. *Support Care Cancer,* Vol.16, No.3 (March 2008), pp. 235-240, ISSN 0941-4355, eISSN 1433-7339.

Sun, Y., Z. Li, M. Sun, L. Chang. (2007). A Study of Attitudes of Family Members of Cancer Patients regarding Truth-Telling and Possible Influencing Factors. *Chinese Journal of Nursing*. No. 6. (in Chinese)

Tang, S. T. and S-Y. C. Lee. (2004). Cancer Diagnosis and Prognosis in Taiwan: patient References versus Experiences. *Psycho-Oncology,* Vol. 13, No.1, (January 2004), pp. 1-13 ISSN: 1057-9249, eISSN 1099-1611.

Tang, S. T. et al. (2008). Patient awareness of prognosis, patient-family caregiver congruence on the preferred place of death, and caregiving burden of families contribute to the equality of life for terminal ill cancer patients in Taiwan. *Psycho-Oncology,* Vol. 17, No. 12, (December 2008), pp.1202-1209, eISSN: 1099-1611.

Tolstoy. L. translated by L. Solotaroff. (1986). *The Death of Ivan Ilyich*. New York: Bantam Book.

Tse, C.Y., A. Chong, and S.Y. Fok. (2003). Breaking Bad News: A Chinese Perspective. *Palliative Medicine* Vol.17, No.4 (June 2003), pp. 339-343, ISSN 0269-2163, eISSN 1477- 030X.

Tuckett. A.G. (2004). Truth-Telling in Clinical Practice and the Arguments For and Against: A Review of Literature. *Nursing Ethics*, Vol.11, No.5, (September 2004), pp. 500-513 ISSN 0969-7330, eISSN 1477-0989.

Wear, S. (2007). Truth Telling to the Sick and Dying in a Traditional Chinese Culture. In S.C. Lee, ed., *The Family, Medical Decision-Making, and Biotechnology*. pp. 71-82 Dordrecht: Springer. ISBN 978-1-4019-5220-4, eISBN 978-1-4020-5220-0, The Netherlands.

Yixue Yu Zhexue (Editorial Office of the journal *Medicine and Philosophy*). (2008). Guiding Principles on Truth-telling to and Consent from Cancer Patients. *Medicine and Philosophy* (Clinical Making Forum Edition) 29 (10): 7-8. (in Chinese)

Zeng, T., Y. Li, Y. Chen, and P. Fang. (2007). An Investigation into the Attitudes of Medical Professional on Disclosing Cancer Diagnoses. *Medicine and Philosophy* (Clinical Decision Making Forum Edition), 28 (11). (in Chinese).

8

Nanotechnology and Ethics: Assessing the Unforeseeable

Monique Pyrrho
University of Brasília
Brazil

1. Introduction

Nanotechnology is not in consensus. The attempts to answer the question "what is nanotechnology?" are usually inaccurate, and the responses to it, far from being unanimous. There has always been controversy, from defining its conception to establishing the limits of the so-called nanoscience subject, as well as its effects and viability. One of the few points of consensus among scientists is that manipulation of materials at the atomic level may unfold new properties.

The emerging nanotechnology brings great excitement due to its technological potential. In order to analyze its possible ethical implications, the task of starting from the beginning, of introducing the theme from the concept of the object of study itself, imposes the first and fundamental obstacle for those who intend to reflect about the ethical approach of nanoscience and nanotechnology.

This initial challenge comes from the differences found between what each group that uses the term nanotechnology intends to mean. The objects of study, nanoscience and nanotechnology do not seem to be consensually organized. In general, researchers and scientists tend to describe nanotechnology from a perspective of their own activities (Petersen & Anderson, 2007).

The prefix nano, derived from the Greek "dwarf", refers to the tiny size of the particles. In scientific terms, it means a part per billion; therefore, a nanometer (nm) corresponds to a billionth of a meter (10^{-9}). To illustrate the reduced scale in which nanotechnology works, the smallest point seen by a human naked eye is about 10,000 nm, while 1 nanometer corresponds to 10 times the diameter of a hydrogen atom (Medeiros et al., 2006).

Under such perspective, it is possible to understand nanoscience as the field of knowledge that studies the fundamental principles of molecules and structures (sized between 1 to 10 nanometers in at least one dimension) called nanostructures. Nanotechnology, in turn, is the application of these nanostructures in functional nanoscale devices.

However, even according to the official definitions by the National Science Foundation (2000), nanotechnology does not have a clear concept. The NSF defines it as the research and technology developed from new properties as a result of matter manipulation on a nanoscale level - between 1 and 100 nm. However, the same properties can be occasionally found in dimensions below 1 nm and above 100 nm.

Nowadays, the manipulation of objects and devices on that scale is common to almost all new fields of experimental science. The difficulty in establishing what is and what is not nanotechnology has important epistemological and ethical consequences (Ferrari, 2010). The ambiguous nature of such concept results in laboratories claiming that their researches must be added the prefix "nano", along with all resources and prestige it brings. The undefined limits of this new techno-scientific movement influence the debate on its potential and its consequences.

Nanotechnology is expected to advance almost all current technological industry branches such as. Literature approaches an expectation of progress in computer science, micro and nanoelectronics, cosmetic and textile industry, energy production and storage, telecommunications, chemical and petrochemical industries, agriculture and agribusiness, automobile industry, aeronautics and, of course, arms industry (Invernizzi, 2008).

As far as healthcare is concerned, nanotechnology shows one of its most promising announcing revolutionary scientific and technological progress that might deeply affect the way we deal with health and medicine in the near future. In the new field of nanomedicine, devices and nanostructured materials are expected to be applied to monitor, repair, build and control human biological systems (Sahoo et al., 2007). There are countless possibilities: controlled release of therapeutic agents, production of active ingredients, medical imaging, lab diagnoses, biomaterial production and implants, and more (Wagner et al., 2006).

The great promises in nanotechnology are not new. The fact that many laboratories are investing more and more in research shows more than a resemblance between nanotechnology and the latest great advances in biotechnology.

Before the promising scientific advances and their impacts come, major social groups have not waited to express their positions on nanotechnology and society. The media, scientists, policymakers and sectors of society have promptly set out their stances, with the justification that scientific changes require urgency in decision-making. A hasty scenario of extreme positions has been set up. However, the shape of this innovation demands balanced reflection rather than taking unconditional sides on the use or ban of nanotechnology, or definitively halting it, or waiting for it to eventually happen. At this initial stage, therefore, it is opportune to propose a prior discussion that is broader than foreknowledge and assessment of the unforeseeable beneficial effects or risks.

As the establishment of the topics for discussion already seems to be difficult strategies other than discussing risks that cannot be fully foreseen and assessed are strongly suggested. This is how this topic will be brought up and developed here.

The first challenge regards the different appropriations of vocabulary and the diversity of devices and techniques used in the various fields of research. This leads to the notion that nanotechnology is not a single entity to which a single value judgment can be attributed. Actually, one should consider not one, but many nanotechnologies. Thus, it would be extremely difficult and also inappropriate to propose a comprehensive stance for all the fields and products involved.

In different scenarios, the term "nanotechnology" can have a different interpretation, eventually being used for different objectives, leading to different consequences. There are some who even question the innovative nature of nanotechnology , grouping it with other fields of biotechnology. This attitude may diminish the hype around this so-called innovation; however, it also points to the need to analyze the various objectives and definitions upon which the debate is based (Ferrari, 2010).

Consequently, instead of mainly establishing concepts and discussing the possible risks related to the use of nanotechnology products, this is a longer and not so explored path.

First of all, there are some important reference points regarding this scientific phenomenon to be defined. Also, innovations in relation to previous biotechnological-scientific advances must be identified, and the degree to which they demand specific debate on their ethics must be assessed.

2. What is new?

In at least one respect, nanotechnology represents something fairly new among technical-scientific revolutions: the ethical implications of its possible discoveries have become a cause for concern even before the discoveries themselves have been made. Indeed, more than the technological advances themselves, what is most innovative in nanotechnology is the very discussion of its ethics, which is taking place at the same time as or before the scientific events on which it focuses. Long before scientists could explore the manipulation and shaping of compounds at atomic and molecular levels, it was the expectation of the transformation of our relationship with the world, of delving so deeply into the structure of matter, which motivated the visionary Feynman (1961) in the first references to the theme. Possible repercussions precede and obscure the actual facts. Debates regarding the possible transformation of the world, and of humans into post-humans, take place before the basic science has been established. Apocalyptic scenarios are depicted even before methods and procedures for nanotechnology can be clearly established (admittedly, this is not unlike some genetics).

Therefore, according to Schummer (2007), the technological exploration of nanoscale properties is not the real innovation. He states that the innovative aspect lies in how nanotechnology and the way it is depicted reflect the connections between society, science and technology. This innovation affects pre-established boundaries between living and non-living things, the natural and the artificial.

It is significant that a debate on ethical implications is taking place before the scientific advances themselves have actually taken place. An ethical approach, rather than an attempt to explore science fiction, could perhaps state that nanoscience, its structures and scientific approaches, represent a characteristic rupture between new paradigms and the classical scientific model.

Innovations frequently disrupt established moral standpoints, bringing discomfort or a conflict between customs and the new reality that is imposed, and requiring further discussion. Moreover, dealing with novelty brings, to some degree, an urge to explore the paths of the unknown which cannot easily be foreseen (Swierstra & Rip, 2007).

In the case of nanotechnology it is characterized not by the size of the particles it deals with but by the new and unknown chemical and physical properties that derive from their size (Ratner & Ratner, 2003). The great attraction of working on a nanoscale lies in new and unusual physical and chemical properties that are not found in the same materials at micro and macroscopic dimensions. It is therefore unrealistic to expect to know all the possibilities for their use and to foresee their consequences. The specific characteristics of the nanometric dimension diverge from the physicochemical laws that determine the behavior of materials at "normal" macroscopic scales.

3. The scientific paradigm and its implications

Given that nanoscience is based on the diverse and unpredicted behaviour of materials manipulated on a nanoscale, the unknown and the unforeseen are central to it. Scientific knowledge, insufficient in itself to provide moral solutions, is also revealed to be incapable of providing sufficiently reliable information to enable proper reflection on the health-related, ecological, ethical and social impacts of nanotechnology.

The literature on nanotechnology and ethics is incipient in comparison with what has been produced internationally regarding its techno-scientific aspects. However, it is noticeable that the ethical implications that have been identified, and the solutions that have been proposed, vary in accordance with the writer's individual perspective on scientific activity.

There is a tendency for scientists to have an inward-looking perspective that describes scientific activity on the basis of its methods and technical results, in this case producing what one might call a scientific image of nanotechnology. The ethical discourse arising from this image emphasizes ethical implications closely connected to the direct consequences of the applications of nanotechnology.

With regard to practical questions regarding health and the expected use of nanomedicine, the ethical issues arising from the applications of nanotechnology are too numerous and complex to be addressed satisfactorily by scientists alone.

If, in the past, the analysis by scientists of ethical issues surrounding technological advances proved to be limited, and sometimes biased, a new science that reveals epistemological ruptures with the fundamental scientific characteristics of reproduction and predictability would appear to present an even more complex subject for analysis.

Another factor to be taken into consideration is that much of the scientific media defines nanoscience not on the basis of its conceptual reference points or properties but in raltion to expectations surrounding its applications. Nanoscience essentially becomes the expectations that are placed upon it, the things it is deemed to promise. This discourse becomes an apology for scientific progress, instead clarifying any specific aspect of nanotechnology (Swierstra & Rip, 2007). Made the object either of huge optimism or huge pessimism, nanotechnology is depicted either as the future solution to world health problems or the future cause of a great ecological disaster. From such a perspective a sensible assessment is impossible.

A new ethical approach is necessary; an approach that uses the language of this new scientific paradigm. It is especially important to know how to engage in dialogue about a science based on the unforeseeable and the unknown.

This ethical debate on nanotechnology highlights the oscillation between the consequentialist and deontological approach, well known in bioethics. The relevance of the consequentialist approach is clear, due to the central role of risk analysis of nanoparticles in this debate (Ferrari, 2010). This is completely understandable since this kind of analysis is necessary in order to guide political and ethical regulation, but it needs to be based on scientific evidence, which is especially problematic in nanotechnology (Shrader-Frechette K, 2007). The discourses on risks become important, partly because current mechanisms for regulation and control are insufficient, sometimes even inadequate, to address the uncertain, unpredictable aspects of this field (Grunwald, 2005).

Those who intend to establish their ethical approach only by studying impacts and detailed risk analyses based on thorough knowledge of technical possibilities, find themselves thwarted. Such failure occurs primarily because scientists' parameters for risks diverge from the perception of such risks within society (Slovic, 1987). The public perception is that biotechnological advances bring unknown risks that may take time to become apparent or may not be fully observable. It is generally opposed to the scientific discourse based on calculations of risks and benefits. But such calculation is not yet possible (and might never be), as the risks and benefits are not yet well known (Savadori et al., 2004). The principle of precaution is frequently presented as a solution to the difficulty of predicting the direction of scientific development. It is seen as a guideline for decisions under uncertain conditions. It is assumed that negative effects are known, but it is impossible to measure risks due to a lack of data (Ferrari, 2010).

Not only is it impossible to measure the risks presented by nanotechnology but even its effects are unpredictable. This is because nanotechnology involves a new epistemic scenario, the inherent basis of which is uncertainty and ignorance (Stirling, 2007). Decision making in nanotechnology, therefore, is additionally complex because of its epistemic nature, as well as other factors such as the wide variety of its applications (Rip, 2006). Consequently, the precautions taken against unknown risks are not successful in practical life and its interactions with the market. The parameters of the analysis therefore need to be revised. The subject has to be analyzed on an interdisciplinary basis, taking into consideration the complexity of the relationships between many levels of reality, and thus encompassing both scientific and social phenomena (Victoriano, 2006). An increasing number of authors criticize risk analysis as the only approach in debates on the ethics of nanotechnology. They suggest that ethical reflections should go beyond risks and benefits to also address the way science is performed, including its objectives and methods. These would be more complete approaches, taking into account issues such as intellectual property, public opinion, and future generations (Ferrari, 2010).

In recent years, especially in Europe, there has been an increasing number of initiatives calling for a more representative inclusion of public opinion in debates on the control and management of new technologies. This movement grew stronger in the wake of negative reactions to foods derived from genetically modified organisms. Such initiatives aim to re-establish trust in science, establish political innovations, avoid adverse reactions, democratize the governance of new technologies, and promote more responsible, reliable scientific practices. However, public engagement can be hampered by many factors: a lack of awareness of what nanotechnology really entails; the future-oriented and promissory character of nanotechnology, which gives a special role to science fiction in shaping the moral imagination of nanoscientists and nanotechnology policy itself; and the very strangeness of nanotechnology in relation to daily life, introducing a dimension that is not well be understood or even perceived. In addition, the conceptions or discourses that guide and define the development of nanotech science, though crucial, vary between the many branches of nanotechnology and different cultural scenarios. Such disharmony makes it necessary to analyze those discourses with the aim of making possible genuine public participation. (Macnaghten, 2010).

An ethical approach, therefore, would mean that nanotechnology is part of a cultural scenario, simultaneously defining and being defined by it. In this way the issue of the different perceptions of the sciences, and the discourses and expectations that surround them, take on great importance, since the way the future is described influences the way it turns out to be. The ethical approach, therefore, needs to be applied to other levels, overcoming precaution and the search for consequences in order to understand science as a thorough phenomenon, in all scientific, cultural, economic and political dimensions (Dupuy & Grinbaum, 2004). Reductionism is no longer acceptable.

One of the possibilities is to understand nanoscience and nanotechnology, with their promising results and unforeseen risks, within a broader context, such as a practical segment of a new scientific paradigm based on its ability to control and manipulate matter at atomic and molecular scales (Kearnes & Macnaghten, 2006).

Kuhn (1962), in The Structure of Scientific Revolutions, described the evolution of modern science and defined scientific paradigms as the successive models on which scientific theories were based. Normal science would mean research based on scientific accomplishments recognized, for a while, as the basis for subsequent practice. Normal science, therefore, would be based on paradigms, i.e. models that structure and order the current stock of scientific knowledge, thereby determining the methods and subjects for study. Paradigms are therefore the basis of normal science, which is generally developed to state and confirm common theories and concepts among scientists.

In the case of the broad field of nanoscience, the paradigm previously applied was known as Newtonian Mechanics. It originated from the Cartesian hypothesis, which in some aspects it advanced and completed, and describes the interactions of macroscopic bodies. The scientific revolution from which the next paradigm will emerge may be structured from current normal science. Therefore normal research, following the Cartesian scientific model for analysis, study and synthesis, has influenced the study of bodies and interactions. The attempts to apply the current paradigm to miniaturization may have brought about its very specific crisis.

The attempts to verify a theoretical paradigm, i.e. the ultimate goal of 'normal science', have detected imperfections and incoherence between theory and phenomena (Kuhn, 1962). The search for the ultimate explanation of the universal law that governs all bodies in their smallest units is halted due to its great divergence from the macroscopic world. At the atomic or molecular level, the laws governing interactions are related to the wave nature of electrons and the frequency and wavelength of their vibrations. Unlike the phenomena predicted by classic scientific theory, the concern of quantum physics is the observation of behavior on a nanometric scale (Ratner & Ratner, 2003).

The appropriation of the scientific paradigm extends beyond the changing of the physical science paradigm. Nanotechnology represents the "convergence of quantum physics, molecular biology, computing science, chemistry and engineering" (Mehta, 2002), and therefore differs from Cartesian scientific knowledge. Whereas the latter seeks specialization, nanotechnology results from a convergence of interdisciplinary concepts, allowing interactions between methods, applications and theoretical foundations in different fields of expertise (Garrafa, 2006).

Such a scenario is close to the current complex scientific paradigms in which interactions transcend conventional divisions between sciences, humanities and biomedicine. Nanoscience thus diverges from the scientific method in which the production of knowledge is based on analysis. Such object-oriented analysis, within scientific practice, has resulted in a disconnection between human sciences and natural sciences (Morin, 1988).

Morin (1988) stated that such a disconnection made it impossible to observe the complex nature of the world, reducing reality to "mathematized" rules and laws that would appear to explain the world perfectly by ignoring unforeseen events or facing them as errors. Reality was seen as the sum of observable phenomena, not taking into consideration the possible overlaps between science and philosophy or between human and biological sciences (Morin, 2008).

Starting from a perception of realities in their full complexity, new technology and a new scientific paradigm have practical implications which go beyond the limits of their original subjects. This complex thinking is illustrated as a network that seeks to analyze the possible interactions between many levels of reality and the repercussions of events. Also, this new thinking includes an awareness that unforeseen events are characteristic of the phenomena; they are not just the result of errors, and are not to be disregarded (Morin, 1988).

From the viewpoint of complexity, the rupture between ecology and sociology, in which scientific analysis has as its object the environment without man and man outside his environment, is artificial and ethnocentric. An analysis of the possible consequences of nanotechnology should, therefore, avoid disconnecting these dimensions (Victoriano, 2006). This is vitally important for a proper analysis of the actual influences and the distribution of social benefits brought about by the minimization of energy and materials required in the nanotechnology industry (Schnaiberg, 2006).

New paradigms generally emerge as more suitable responses to questions unanswered by previous paradigms. They enable scientists to explain a greater number of phenomena or to increase the accuracy of their existing explanations. For this reason the application of new technologies may be controversial, because they might seem to offer a theoretical solution to the world's problems, and because they unveil a set of unknown phenomena that might be greeted with disbelief or sometimes even panic (Kuhn, 1962).

Nanotechnology is paradigmatic in this sense. Sometimes it is portrayed as a revolutionary technology that will change the way we live through its effects on industry, communications and information technology. It would appear to expand the boundaries of medicine, promising less invasive, more effective surgery, more specific medications, treatments for incurable diseases such as cancer, and even the possibility of improvements in cognition and memory processes (Freitas, 2005).

On the other hand, the current lack of knowledge regarding the potential scope of nanotechnology provokes extreme reactions that tend to emphasize environmental risks and profound transformations in our way of life. One example is the debate on the so-called "grey goo", a scenario where self-replicating nanoscale devices called nanobots would rule the world. Out of human control, they would eventually eliminate our species from the planet (Drexler, 2004).

The advances within nanotechnology have led to debates on the ethical implications of its applications. The ethical issues discussed have included equity, benefit distribution, access to scientific advances, environmental impact (the use of new materials, and of new properties of previously-known materials, might make them insoluble or turn them into pollutants), implications for privacy and security (invisible surveillance equipment, and infinite possibilities for the arms industry), modification of the constitution of living entities (genetically modified organisms), and self-replicating devices (Salvarezza, 2003).

In its methods and in the way it is conceived, managed and practiced, the new scientific paradigm of nanotechnology represents a rupture with the existing scientific model. The current academic scientific model, conceived in 18th-century Europe, especially in French and German universities, has been undergoing profound transformations. Post-academic science shares the objectives of the previous model - the production of knowledge in accordance with epistemic norms, scientific laws, and values - and yet differs from it in at least three aspects: how knowledge is produced (focusing on transdisciplinarity); how knowledge is assessed (for its economic potentials); and the great emphasis on the application of that knowledge, or in other words, the fact that knowledge is produced so as to serve certain technological purposes (Jotterand, 2005).

The common perception of nanotechnology as a revolution is therefore understandable. Nanotechnology not only entails epistemic rupture, as did the other scientific revolutions before it, but introduces new laws and structures of knowledge, or new cognitive categories. Changing the way categories are explained brings changes to the way we experience the world.

Nanotechnology, however, is more than a scientific revolution; it is probably a techno-scientific revolution, because it focuses not on the properties of matter but on its manipulation and transformation.

Therefore, in a way that is quite revolutionary, neither the concept of science nor the concept of technology can perfectly describe the know-how of nanotechnology. Nordmann (2004) states that nanoscience is not structured from a topic but set to a goal. It is not aimed at manifestations of nature, machines, or substances with new properties. Its epistemic effectiveness is not measured based on its devices and the functions of substances. Actually, nanoscience is an attempt to explore an inhospitable territory and to colonize a new world, or an as-yet unexplored area of the world. Epistemic success is now a technical accomplishment; the ability to act in nanoscale scenarios, to see, to move things, to carve a word in a molecule. This means that nanoscience is not traditional "science" per se, and that there is no distinction between its theoretical manifestation and its technical intervention, or between the understanding of nature and its transformation. From now on, therefore, it would be more appropriate for the debate to be focused on nanotechnoscience.

This particular scenario of technoscientific revolution does not only establish nanotechnology's scientific and technological development, but also influences the development of moral reflections on the social and ethical implications of nanotechnology. The technoscientific revolution brought about by nanotechnoscience is a broader post-academic scientific movement in which science, technology, politics and economics have convergent social purposes. These relationships allow greater integration between ethical and philosophical reflections and scientific practice within the post-academic context, due to its cross-disciplinary nature and to the increasing political and social pressure on the process of scientific knowledge production (Jotterand, 2005).

Sotolongo (2006) pointed out two important ethical issues that require closer attention, both relate to the current type of science exemplified in nanoscience. First, due to humans' great capacity to intervene in natural phenomena, and unprecedented capacity to interact with and manipulate matter and energy, our physical and intellectual abilities can be enhanced through autonomous integrated systems. The closer science comes to controlling environmental conditions, the closer it gets to potential powers of destruction. The second issue is the huge extent of the knowledge acquired, which makes it impossible to identify all the possible uses and practical interactions of the resulting technologies. As far as natural and social complexity is concerned, not all the practical implications can be known, predicted or manipulated: on the contrary, there is an inherent uncertainty in the implications.

Although many adverse results can be expected in relation to nanotechnology, not restricted to the immediate threat of nanotoxicity to humans, it is a cause for concern that so few studies of its ethical, environmental, political and social implications have been carried out. Even though there was reflection on its potential impacts before nanotechnology entered scientific practice, the fast growth of research in its technical and scientific aspects over recent years contrasts with the lack of investment and scientific production with regard to its ethical and social aspects. Indeed, there has been an increasing distance between the expanding technical-scientific knowledge and the required socio-political and philosophical reflections (Mnyusiwalla et al., 2003).

The convergence of effort and investment in the technical fields is clearly related to the social representation of science: the cultural phenomenon in which interpretive science, which seeks meanings, loses out to empirical science, which seeks laws and rules (Franklin, 1995).

Faced with the innovation and the amount of challenges posed by the ethical debate on nanotechnology, there are those who propose nanoethics, a subject that would be devoted exclusively to the analysis of these challenges. However, immediate questions arise about whether an area of ethical study devoted exclusively to nanotechnology is really necessary. Consequently, comparisons between bioethics and nanoethics are frequently made. Nanotechnology does not demand a genuinely new ethical approach but instead an approach that is different and renewed in relation repertoire of the previous ones. Therefore, instead of declaring that these questions have already been asked and that there is nothing new in nanotechnology, it can be pointed out that if the questions are the same ones as before, it is because they have not yet been answered. It is worthwhile to pose those same questions again, for they might help to elucidate the phenomenon (Khushf, 2007).

The same answers and methods that did not completely illustrate the analyzed phenomenon are dispensable, therefore, but not the ethical concern itself. As previously suggested, the development of nanotechnology casts doubt on whether risk assessments and other analyses that are commonly used will nowadays suffice when it comes to evaluating nanotechnology. Although traditional ethical approaches can be appropriate for some subjects, nanotechnoscience has social and ethical implications of such magnitude that it necessitates the development of alternative approaches that can provide conditions for the development of nanotechnology (Meaney, 2006).

Therefore, whether proceeding from the perspective of nanoethics or from that of other disciplines, the discussion regarding the ethical implications of nanotechnology reveals that the questions do not arise only from within the social sciences: the scientists start to question their own practices.

Despite manifesting this initial interest in reflecting upon their practices, the discourses of natural science and social sciences are not the same. This is due especially to two factors. First, following the events of World War II, scientists acquired a greater sensitivity to their technological impacts. This sensibility focuses mainly on the impact of devices, concentrating concerns on environmental and health issues. Another factor that sets their discourses apart is the different readership for natural science articles when compared with the social sciences and humanities.

4. Some ethical approaches: A typology

The purpose of setting the scenario in which nanotechnology has been established is to show how the concepts of nanotechnology and the corresponding moral considerations of the different actors, including scientists, are heterogeneous. The proposed approach, therefore, starts from this initial effort to identify the concepts, their origins and their effects (Kaiser, 2006).

Aiming to avoid the dualism that is so prevalent nowadays, Kaiser (2006) suggested that the strategy for avoiding utopia or dystopia in the debate was to adopt an observational stance, rather than viewing ethics from a participative perspective. According to him, it would not be necessary to define nanotechnology, given its uncertain and unpredictable nature, in order to conduct a debate on it. The strategy suggested would be to stand back from the topic and observe the scenario within which the actors construct their perspectives on and concepts of nanotechnology, in order, to guide the ethical analysis.

Grunwald (2005), for instance, argues that the innovative character of nanotechnology is being overestimated and that the ethical analysis should focus on the various representations that underlie the discussion. It is not the nanoscale and its processes that have ethical and social consequences. Ethical reflection should embrace science as part of human relationships, with their images, significances and expectations.

Accordingly, to understand technologies in order to develop an appropriate ethical approach, it is necessary to have explored in detail the universe of visions, images, ideas and representations of nature, and of the human being embedded in the discussion (Ferrari, 2010). This perspective relates to the argument of the philosopher Karl Popper, who states that every scientific theory is based on a set of values and world views. Roughly speaking, those world views make up what he calls a Metaphysical Research Program. They are not susceptible to direct empirical testing and are not falsifiable, and do not properly constitute scientific knowledge, but they determine which problems, investigation methods and solutions are considered scientifically (Popper, 2009).

Dupuy (2006) states that in nanotechnology, as in other convergence technologies, the Metaphysical Research Program is characterized by a lack of distinction between knowing and doing. Such similarity, which seems to reach its peak in nanotechnology, is illustrated precisely by the instruments that make it technically possible.

In 1981, the Scanning Tunneling Microscope was developed. Through a very thin tip and a voltage bias, it allowed atomic dimensions and dispositions to be analyzed, and it was later discovered that this same instrument, with a small modification, was capable of manipulating and repositioning atoms very accurately (Cao, 2006).

Dupuy (2006) argues that the Metaphysical Research Program goes beyond this very explanatory metaphor of the microscope. Nanotechnology would make possible the engineering of evolution, enabling man to be the designer in the production of life. According to Dupuy, a project of such magnitude could not be analyzed using pre-established ethical doctrines. A new ethical challenge requires a meticulous exercise of unveiling the conceptions, ideas and images on which the scientific theory is based, so as to then proceed to a critical analysis or a normative judgment of the technological progress.

In reply to the question "what is science?" different answers are given, but all of them are always set in a certain context. The different forms of interpreting this question give birth to at least two different images of science.

Dealing with different representations of science, Olivé (2006) stated that both the "scientific image" and the "philosophical image" of science are derived from the question "What is science?". While the "scientific image" is usually the way in which scientists describe their own activities, the "philosophical image" seeks to characterize scientific production within the contexts provided.

The "scientific image" is to describes scientific facts and elucidates the rules governing patterns, without concern for the social criticism of its own process of knowledge construction (Franklin, 1995). The "philosophical image" studies the history, sociology and philosophy of science and relates scientific activities to social practices and institutions, to the conditions for the development of science, and to the mutual repercussions of society and science (Olivé, 2006).

It is not specifically the dimension of the nanoparticles, therefore, that is important for studies and consequent debates on the interactions between technology and society. The analysis depends on the views of nanotechnology held by the different actors. What matters is the transformation after human interference, and not the nanometric dimension in itself, given that such a dimension is found in nature regardless of the intervention by human devices. It is emphasized, however, that no intrinsic moral value is derived from human intervention. Whether or not one carbon compound is nanostructured does not make it ethically superior to another. It is in the relations between men, in society, and as part of the natural environment, that the products and their uses will be revealed as more or less adequate.

Some of the ethical implications therefore seem to be clearly demonstrated, such as in the example of a compound that is toxic or pollutes. Other ethical challenges become clear only within complex social interactions, such as the repercussions for the global economy and the social inequality resulting from the introduction and appropriation of nanotechnologies by the market.

Assuming that the ethical approach towards nanotechnology starts from the paradigmatic unpredictability of this technical-scientific phenomenon, a schematic consideration of the possible questions is put forward here. The dilemmas resulting from the interaction between a new scientific paradigm and the complex overall social dynamics, together with the image of nanoscience on which the ethical perspective is based, produce a classification scheme for the implications of nanotechnology that has two categories: autogenous (internal) and heterogeneous (external) (Pyrrho, 2008).

4.1 Autogenous ethical implications

Nanotechnologies are characteristically improvement technologies, which is to say that like many convergence technologies, they refine and improve tools and materials that will be used in other fields. They not only change the existing components and devices but also develop new ones. This is the aspect most closely related to scientifically observable consequences, which sometimes have considerable implications. Although nanoparticles are not present-day inventions, the capacity to structure them systematically for the industrial exploitation of their properties is certainly new. Products developed this way for sporting, nutritive, automotive, cosmetic, information technological and many other purposes are now available on the market. This production on an industrial scale is critical because it may cause significant damage to the environment, to workers, and to the large populations that are eager for technological goods.

The partial lack of knowledge about the properties of the materials goes together with the way in which the national and international regulatory bodies lag behind: the regulations take the chemical composition of the components into account but not their conformation. For example, it is possible for a new nanostructured component to arrive on the pharmaceutical market without undergoing new toxicity tests, even though the reactions within the organism may be completely different.

Such developments are usually accompanied by biased arguments characterized by an assumption that the application of nanotechnology is inevitable, a fascination regarding its implementation, and a reduction of the ethical debate to the analysis of toxicological and environmental risks. The perspective of those making such arguments is that the benefits from research are usually derived more or less automatically, that any negative effects can be attributed to mistakes on the part of others, and that it is impossible to predict how technology will be used once it has been developed (Ferrari, 2010). This perspective clearly attributes moral neutrality to science. Risks and negative effects are external to the scientific activity, so it cannot be responsible for them. This view also produces a common perspective in bioethical discourse – the search for technical solutions for moral problems.

According to Schummer (2004), three different understandings of the "social and ethical implications of nanotechnology" stand out among scientists. Computer sciences researchers associate these implications with radical changes in society, in which everything is possible with software programming. Natural science researchers seem to hold a more modest but still visionary position about industrial revolutions and other deep changes, as in biomedical practices that related to nanotechnology. For toxicologists and environmentalists, meanwhile, the ethical and social implications represent risks for health and for the environment.

Despite the common ignorance regarding nanotechnology and its risks, the scientific image seems to result in a positive perspective on the impacts of nanotechnology. In another study, based on interviews with researchers, many of the interviewees emphasized the difficulty in analyzing the risks due to the lack of research and knowledge regarding important aspects of the nanomaterials. They pointed out difficulties in foreseeing the behavior of the particles in certain environments, the little investment in risk analyses, and uncertainty regarding current methods of risk analysis for the nanoparticles. They described nanoscience as currently going through a latency period between the introduction of the technologies and the evaluation of the adverse effects. They still took the view, however, that nanotechnology is positive for society (Petersen & Anderson, 2007).

The autogenous ethical implications were not highlighted because of an understanding that they are intrinsic to nanotechnology. Such a view could erroneously put value on the applications of this technology. The implications are considered autogenous as they are associated with a causal effect. These are implications that are conceptualized within the technical perspective. They generally result from the application of such approaches, without complex analysis of interference from other factors. They are the repercussions that are most frequently mentioned in debates since they are close to the predominant ethical model of science, which is usually limited to assessing the impact of products and devices on the environment and on health. However, at the point where such use seems to present risks that are more measurable and analyzable, it has to be ensured that the same technology that enables it is capable of supplying instruments that are sufficiently accurate to assess any failures and to propose solutions (Pyrrho, 2008).

4.2 Heterogenous ethical implications

The term heterogeneous refers to the fact that studies on nanotechnological devices and their implications are conceived through different "images" of science. While the devices result from the "scientific image", the social understanding of their use relates to a "meta-scientific" perspective on nanotechnology.

The possible repercussions from the use of nanotechnology that are dealt with here arise from interfaces of various cultural, social, economic, environmental and political dimensions. They are heterogeneous because they result from complex interactions and not from evaluations performed by science itself. They require an ethical assessment that diverges from the search for cause-effect relationships and consequent linear risk analyses (Pyrrho, 2008).

Expectations of technical solutions for social problems, such as the prospect that some of the main applications of nanotechnology could make it easier to achieve the United Nations Development Targets through energy production and increased agricultural productivity (Salamanca-Buentello et al., 2005), have raised environmental, political, economic and public health questions that, due to their mutual implications, trigger a discussion that does not deal in simple solutions.

There is quite a widespread understanding that nanotechnology represents a technological revolution that poses new challenges for traditional understandings about science and knowledge acquisition, its intrinsically unpredictable character serving to question the role of science in searching for truth. The new facets that science has been acquiring are dictated strongly by the avidity of the market for technology. This process through which science is transformed into techno-science is followed by reconfigurations of economic power, and consequently also of political power. This politicization of science, and of nanotechnology specifically, which represents the convergence of science, technology, politics and economy for social and government purposes, offers the possibility of a better integration of ethical and philosophical reflections with scientific and technological development (Jotterand, 2006).

This type of analysis emphasizes nanotechnology as a social-technical system and the cultural values infused in the technologies. The social scientists and ethical consultants who devote themselves to the study of nanotechnology can therefore influence nanotechnology, together with other actors. As a consequence, when understanding nanotechnology as an emerging technology, it is important to address the systems/networks of people and things. While the technology is being developed, the distribution of power and authority is being built, meanings are being contested and consolidated, and social practices involving rights and responsibilities are being established. These social arrangements are a subject that should be examined in the light of ethics, using ethical concepts, language, principles, norms and theories (Johnson, 2007).

In the philosophical image of nanotechnology there is a predominant criticism of the so-called nanohype and of the dualist and reductionist discussion to which it has led. The dystopian and utopian visions frequently provoke extreme reactions: the former frequently produce widespread rejection while the latter often lead to eventual disappointment at the gap between expectations and reality, as in the case of genetically modified organisms. There is a strong suggestion that social engagement take place in an effective way and not only as a form of avoiding public non-acceptance.

Although some heterogeneous ethical implications such as social control, intellectual property, the knowledge economy and social (in)justice have not attracted media or public attention in the way that cinematographic cyborgs and promised panaceas have done, the implications that are often forgotten are the ones that portray the most tangible and important dimensions for an analysis of ethics in nanotechnology.

While recognizing the possibility of problems in classification, the categories proposed here can highlight possibilities for evaluating risks resulting from nanotechnology and the complex interdependencies that are socially related. The categories point towards social dynamics as the locus where diverse ethical reflections and public debates are increasingly necessary.

5. Conclusion

The challenging character of nanotechnology is illustrated by its cross-disciplinary nature and the impossibility of ascertaining all of its applications and implications. Even the theoretical foundations of nanoscience are based on these innovative features. The unfeasibility of attaining this overall knowledge of nanotechnology, and the unpredictability inherent in the properties it explores, are responsible not only for the emergence of new ethical challenges but also for the need for a diverse approach.

It is clear that there can be a distinction between traditional ethics, which seeks answers to questions already posed, and a conception that attempts ethical reflections regarding the possible moral implications of the application of this new technology. This difference, together with an understanding of the complexity of reality, indicates that there is a need for an innovative kind of analysis. Therefore, to debate and eventually come up with moral answers regarding nanotechnology, it is necessary to have a perspective with a sufficiently dynamic basis that is not limited to a strictly codified ethics.

The approach needed to analyze an emerging technology is one that considers not only the complexity of reality as a whole but also specific moral questions of a given socio-cultural context. Consequently, the ethical values required are no longer those that are based epistemologically on principles that lack both a sufficiently stratified theoretical basis and applicability in complex contexts. They must not be based on accumulated segmented scientific knowledge but on knowledge (of the facts) that considers complexity. From this it is may be possible to generate normative implications that are applicable to a moral dialogue that is guided by tolerance to differences and may also point toward decisions in different socioeconomic and cultural situations.

Far from attributing intrinsic moral values, the intention in proposing a distinction between autogenous and heterogeneous implications for the construction of an ethical approach towards nanotechnology, taking into account the fallibility to which all classifications are subject, is to distinguish these perspectives from the interactions that this approach addresses.

The processes of research, production and application of nanotechnology are approached as autogenous themes. Ethical reflections that involve risk analysis, which is not always possible, demand a double ability: technical improvement, with the development of adequate devices for such evaluations, and also the search for new ethical considerations that are sustained even if knowledge is not imminently attained.

The heterogeneous questions, which deal with the complex interactions of society, technology, environment, politics and economics, within the still incipient discussion on the ethics of nanotechnology, are the ones that have received least attention, even though a sober and attentive reading shows that they are extremely relevant and plausible.

In the light of the hype driving the race between laboratories to label their research with the prefix "nano", and between countries to lead the way in producing state-of-the-art nanotechnology, political agents oscillate between disregarding ethical matters and calling for a definitive moratorium on research. Given this scenario, ethical reflection on the subject of nanotechnology has to be free from overreaction and immediacy. The approach taken toward the emerging technologies, as in the case of nanotechnology, should sober, critical and dialectical. A diversity of perspectives and interests should be considered when searching for answers to the ethical challenges imposed by nanotechnology in the complex modern context.

6. Acknowledgment

This work would not have been possible without the services of the University of Brasilia Central Library.
Thanks also to Dr. Gabriele Cornelli for his unselfish and unfailing support.

7. References

Cao, G. (2006). *Nanostructures & Nanomaterials: Synthesis, Properties & Applications*, Imperial College Press, ISBN 978-981-4322-50-8, London, United Kingdom

Drexler, E.K. (2004). Nanotechnology: From Feynman to Funding. *Bulletin of Science, Technology & Society*, Vol. 24, No. 1, (February 2004), pp. 21-27, ISSN 0270-4676.

Dupuy, J-P. & Grinbaum, A. (2004). Living with Uncertainty: Toward the Ongoing Normative Assessment of Nanotechnology. *Techné*, Vol. 8, No. 2, (December - March 2004), pp. 4–25, ISSN 1091-9264.

Dupuy, J-P. (2006). Les Défis Éthiques des Nanotechnologies. *Science & Devenir de l'Homme : Les Cahiers du MURS*, No. 47, (January-March 2006), pp. 53-67, ISSN 1950-4527.

Ferrari, A. (2010). Developments in the Debate on Nanoethics: Traditional Approaches and the Need for New Kinds of Analysis. *Nanoethics*, Vol. 4, No. 1, (April 2010), pp. 27-52, ISSN 1871-4757.

Feynman, R.P. (1961). There's Plenty of Room at the Bottom. In: *Miniaturization*, Gilbert, H.D., pp. 282-296, Reinhold Publishing Corporation, ISBN 978-027-8919-12-9, New York, United States of America.

Franklin, S. (1995). Science as Culture, Culture of Science. *Annual Review of Anthropology*, Vol. 24, (October 1995), pp. 163-84, ISSN 0084-6570.

Freitas, R.A. (2005). What is Nanomedicine? *Nanomedicine, Nanotechnology, Biology and Medicine*, Vol. 1, No. 1, (March 2005), pp. 2-9, ISSN 1549-9634.

Garrafa, V. (2006). Multi-inter-transdisciplinaridade, complexidade e totalidade concreta em Bioética. In: *Bases Conceituais da Bioética: Enfoque Latino-Americano*, Garrafa, V.; Kottow, M. & Saada, A., pp. 73-85, Gaia, ISBN 85-7555-077-2, São Paulo, Brazil.

Grunwald, A. (2005). Nanotechnology – a New Field of Ethical Enquiry? *Science and Engineering Ethics*, Vol. 11, No. 2, (April 2005), pp. 187–201, ISSN 1353-3452.

Invernizzi, N. (2008). Visions of brazilian scientists on nanosciences and nanotechnologies. *Nanoethics*, Vol. 2, No. 2, (August 2008), pp. 133-148, ISSN 1871-4757.

Johnson, D.G. (2007). Ethics and Technology 'in the Making': an Essay on the Challenge of Nanoethics. *NanoEthics*, Vol. 1, No. 1, (March 2007), pp. 21-30, ISSN 1871-4757.

Jotterand, F. (2005). *Nanotechnology, Bioethics and the Techno-Scientific Revolution: Philosophical and Ethical Assessment of Nanotechnology and Its Applications in Medicine* [PhD Thesis], Rice University, Houston, United States of America.

Jotterand, F. (2006). The Politicization of Science and Technology: Its Implications for Nanotechnology. *Journal of Law, Medicine and Ethics*, Vol. 34, No. 4, (December - March 2006), pp. 658-666, ISSN 1748-720x.

Kaiser, M. (2006). Drawing the Boundaries of Nanoscience: Rationalizing the Concerns? *Journal of Law, Medicine and Ethics*, Vol. 34, No. 4, (December - March 2006), pp. 667-674, ISSN 1748-720x.

Kearnes, M. & Macnaghten, P. (2006). ``Re-imagining Nanotechnology''. *Science as Culture*, Vol. 15, No. 4, (December 2006), pp. 279- 290, ISSN 1470-1189.

Khushf, G. (2007). Open Questions in the Ethics of Convergence. *Journal of Medicine and Philosophy*, Vol. 32, No. 3, (June 2007), pp. 299 - 310, ISSN 1744-5019.

Kuhn, T.S. (1962). *The Structure of Scientific Revolutions*, University of Chicago Press, ISBN 978-022-645-808-3, Chicago, United States of America.

Macnaghten, P. (2010). Researching Technoscientific Concerns in the Making: Narrative Structures, Public Responses, and Emerging Nanotechnologies. *Environment and Planning A*, Vol. 42, No. 1, (January 2010), pp. 23- 37, ISSN 1472-3409.

Meaney, M.E. (2006). Lessons from the Sustainability Movement - Toward an Integrative Decision-Making. *The Journal of Law, Medicine & Ethics*, Vol. 34, No. 4, (December - March 2006), pp. 682-688, ISSN 1748-720x.

Medeiros, E.S.; Paterno, L.G. & Mattoso, L.H.C. (2006). Nanotecnologia. In: *Nanotecnologia: Introdução, Preparação e Caracterização de Nanomateriais e Exemplos de Aplicação*, Durán, N.; Mattoso, L.H.C. & Morais, P.C., pp.14-29, Artliber, ISBN 978-858-8098-336, São Paulo, Brazil.

Mehta, M. (2002). Nanoscience and Nanotechnology: Assessing the Nature of Innovation in these Fields. *Bulletin of science, technology & Society*, Vol. 22, No. 4, (August 2002), pp. pp. 269-273, ISSN 0270-4676.

Mnyusiwalla, A.; Daar, A.S. & Singer, P.A. (2003). 'Mind the Gap': Science and Ethics in Nanotechnology. *Nanotechnology*, Vol. 14, No. 3, (March 2003), pp. R9-R13, ISSN 1361-6528.

Morin, E. (1988). Le Défi de la Complexité. *Revue Chimères*, No. 5-6, pp. 79-94, ISSN 0986-6035.

Morin, E. (2008). Blind Intelligence. In: *On Complexity*, Morin, E., pp. 1-5, Hampton Press, ISBN 978-157-2738-010, New Jersey, United States of America.

National Science Foundation (NSF). (2000). Nanotechnology Definition, In: *National Science Foundation*, March 30, 2010, Avaiable from:
<http://www.nsf.gov/crssprgm/nano/reports/omb_nifty50.jsp>

Nordmann, A. (2004). Molecular Disjunctions: Staking Claims at the Nanoscale. In: *Discovering the Nanoscale*, Baird, D.; Nordmann, A. & Schummer, J. (Eds.), pp. 51-55, IOS Press, ISBN 978-158-6034-672, Amsterdam, Netherlands.

Olivé, L. (2006). *El Bien, el Mal y la Razón: Facetas de la Ciencia y de la Tecnologia*, Paidós, ISBN 978-968-8534-533, Mexico City, Mexico.

Petersen, A. & Anderson, A. (2007). A Question of Balance or Blind Faith? Scientists and Science Policymakers Representations of the Benefits and Risks of anotechnologies. *NanoEthics*, Vol. 1, No. 3, (December 2007), pp. 243-256, ISSN 1871-4757.

Popper, K. (2009). Darwinism as a Metaphysical Research Programme. In: *Philosophy After Darwin: Classic and Contemporary Readings*, Ruse, M., pp. 167-174, Princeton University Press, ISBN 978-0691135540, Princeton, United States of America.

Pyrrho, M. (2008). Nanociência e Bioética: Novas Abordagens Éticas para Novos Paradigmas Científicos. *Revista Brasileira de Bioética,* Vol. 4, No. 3-4, (October - December 2008), pp. 222-235, ISSN 1808-6020.

Ratner, M. & Ratner, D. (2003). *Nanotechnology: a Gentle Introduction to the Next Big Idea,* Prentice Hall, ISBN 978-013-1014-008, New Jersey, United States of America.

Rip, A. (2006). Folk Theories of Nanotechnologists. *Science as Culture,* Vol. 15, No. 4, (December 2006), pp. 349- 365, ISSN 1470-1189.

Sahoo, S.K.; Parveen, S. & Panda, J.J. (2007). The Present and the Future of Nanotechnology in Human Health Care. *Nanomedicine, Nanotechnology, Biology and Medicine,* Vol. 3, No. 1, (March 2007), pp. 20-31, ISSN 1549-9634.

Salamanca-Buentello, F.; Persad, D.L.; Court, E.B.; Martin, D.K.; Daar, A.S. & Singer, P.A. (2005). Nanotechnology and the Developing World. *Plos Medicine,* Vol. 2, No. 5, (May 2005), pp. 383-386, ISSN 1549-1676.

Salvarezza, R.C. (2003). Why is Nanotechnology Important for Developing Countries? *Proceedings of the Third Session of the World Commission on the Ethics of Scientific Knowledge and Technology,* Rio de Janeiro, Brazil, December 2003, pp. 134-36, Avaible from: < http://unesdoc.unesco.org/images/0013/001343/134391e.pdf>

Savadori, L.; Savio, S.; Nicotra, E.; Rumiati, R.; Finucane, M. & Slovic, P. (2004). Expert and Public Perception of Risk from Biotechnology. *Risk Analysis,* Vol. 24, No. 5, (October 2004), pp. 1289-1299, ISSN 1573-9147.

Schnaiberg, A. (2006). Contradições nos Futuros Impactos Socioambientais Oriundos da Nanotecnologia. In: *Nanotecnologia, Sociedade e Meio-ambiente,* Martins, P.R.(org.), pp. 79-86, Xamã, ISBN 85-7587-056-4 , São Paulo, Brazil.

Schummer, J (2004). "Societal and Ethical Implications of Nanotechnology": Meanings, Interest Groups, and Social Dynamics. *Techné,* Vol. 8, No. 2, (December - March 2004), pp. 56-87, ISSN 1091-9264.

Schummer, J. (2007). Identifying Ethical Issues of Nanotechnologies. In: *Nanotechnologies, Ethics and Politics,* Ten Have, H.A.M.J. (ed.), pp. 79–98, UNESCO Publishing, ISBN 978-923-1040-511, Paris, France.

Shrader-Frechette, K. (2007). Nanotoxicology and Ethical Conditions for Informed Consent. *Nanoethics,* Vol. 1, No. 1, (March 2007), pp. 47-56, ISSN 1871-4757

Slovic, P. (1987). Perception of Risk. *Science,* Vol. 236, No. 4799, (April 1987), pp. 280-286, ISSN 1095-9203.

Sotolongo, P.L. (2006). O Tema da Complexidade no Contexto da Bioética. In: *Bases Conceituais da Bioética: Enfoque Latino-Americano,* Garrafa, V.; Kottow, M. & Saada, A., pp. 93-113, Gaia, ISBN 85-7555-077-2, São Paulo, Brazil.

Stirling, A. (2007) Risk, Precaution and Science: Towards a More Constructive Policy. *EMBO Reports,* Vol. 8, No. 4, (April 2007), pp. 309–315, ISSN 1469-3178.

Swierstra, T. & Rip, A. (2007). Nano-Ethics as NEST-Ethics: Patterns of Moral Argumentation About New and Emerging Science and Technology. *NanoEthics,* Vol. 1, No. 1, (March 2007), pp. 3-20, ISSN 1871-4757.

Victoriano, J.M.R. (2006). Intersecções entre Sociologia e Ecologia: a Pesquisa como Fenômeno Social Total a partir da Perspectiva Crítica de Jesús Ibáñez. In:

Nanotecnologia, Sociedade e Meio-ambiente, Martins, P.R.(org.), pp. 87-109, Xamã, ISBN 85-7587-056-4 , São Paulo, Brazil.

Wagner, V.; Dullaart, A.; Bock, A-K. & Zweck, A. (2006). The Emerging Nanomedicine Landscape. *Nature Biotechnology,* Vol. 24, No. 10 (October 2006), pp.1211-1217, ISSN 1546-1696.

9

Speculative Ethics: Valid Enterprise or Tragic Cul-De-Sac?

Michael King, Maja Whitaker and Gareth Jones
Bioethics Centre and Department of Anatomy, University of Otago
New Zealand

1. Introduction

The excitement generated by major scientific advances almost inevitably leads to intense speculation concerning the uses to which these advances will be put. Since some of these will be accompanied by ethical challenges, it is appropriate for bioethicists to delve into their potential ethical implications. If the ethical dimensions of such advances can be outlined and analyzed in advance, this would appear to be a welcome contribution to any public debate that may ensue. However, the speculations range from those that could eventuate within the near future and would represent an incremental change to present practices, to those that are vastly less likely to come to pass and predict paradigmatic shifts of momentous proportions. The challenge for bioethicists is to determine whether they should devote their attention to such extreme speculative possibilities, or to more circumscribed speculations, or indeed whether it is better to focus on existing issues, rather than those that are merely possible.

An illustration of more circumscribed speculation is provided by no less a scientific authority than Francis Collins in his 1999 Shattuck Lecture, in which he speculated on the medical and societal consequences of the Human Genome Project in 2010, just 11 years into the future. He described this as a hypothetical clinical encounter in which a 23-year-old undergoes a battery of genetic tests. This was because by 2010 Collins speculated that the field of pharmacogenetics would have blossomed to such an extent that a prophylactic drug regimen based on personal genetic data could be prescribed to reduce cholesterol level and the risk of coronary artery disease (Collins, 1999). As we look back at 2010 we can see that these goals have not as yet been realized at the level hypothesized by Collins. The question then is whether bioethical enquiry into the prospects opened up by genomic medicine has been weakened by this excessive optimism.

Interestingly, at much the same time, Holtzman and Marteau (2000) contended that the new genetics would not revolutionize the way in which common diseases are identified or prevented. In wanting people to see beyond the genetic hype, they pointed to the importance of existing issues, such as social structures, lifestyle and environment, for much of disease. They also questioned how much interest would be shown in being tested genetically and even more in making appropriate lifestyle choices. These too are considerations calling for the attention of bioethicists.

It is evident then that even relatively focused speculation has its problems. What about far more exploratory and aggressive speculation? Garreau (2005) considers that we are at a turning point in history since our technologies are now capable of altering our minds, memories, metabolisms, personalities and progeny, and similar conjectures motivate Bailey's (2005) "liberation biology". Such vistas have led serious scholars to devote considerable effort towards counteracting what they see as a dangerous drift towards human self-modification, genetic perfectibility and eugenic aspirations (Habermas, 2003). The end-result of these biomedical technologies, it is claimed, is the emergence of programmed people, epitomized by lack of moral responsibility since they are no longer the authors of their own selves. These concerns emanate directly from taking seriously highly speculative futuristic visions of medical accomplishments and often conflating these with current reality.

The question we are addressing here is whether bioethicists should spend time and effort on speculative possibilities like these. In this chapter we describe and analyze some areas of applied ethics (particularly bioethics) in which speculation is at its most adventurous, such as nanotechnology, genetic technology, regenerative medicine, and cryonics. Possibly the most speculative of these is cryonics, which draws on the rest as potential means for fulfilling its vision. Because of these qualities, cryonics will be explored in greater depth as a case study in speculative ethics.

The technologies underlying these areas require ethical attention and analysis; they deliver new abilities into the hands of those who seek to use them, and ethical reflection helps to determine the nature and extent of use that can be defended as being responsible. There may be instances where this leads to a call for a prohibition on the use of a particular technology, as has been the case of genetic engineering. Further, a new technology can have unintended consequences that ethical scrutiny can help to reveal and evaluate.

In evaluating new and emerging technologies one of the major problems is arriving at an understanding of what the technologies are, and of how they might be developed in the future. This, as we have seen, is a path beset by uncertainties, yet understanding them as much as possible is integral to informing moral evaluation of them. This is because judgments that rely on false beliefs about new technologies can have pernicious consequences for the use of the technologies, and for the credibility of applied ethics. As speculation becomes more radical, and our uncertainty about the prediction increases, the epistemic status of applied ethics becomes less secure, and its value more questionable. To explore these issues, we address arguments for and against the role of speculation in ethical analysis of technology, and suggest some boundaries on ethical engagement with speculative matters. First, we will survey some areas of science and technology, focusing on the role that speculation has played in their development.

2. Genomic medicine

Genetics has to some degree always played a role in modern health care, but it was thought that the decoding of the human genome in 2003 would provide unprecedented understanding of the functions and interactions of the entire genome, producing a revolution in health care under the rubric of genomic medicine (Guttmacher and Collins, 2002). It was hoped that a clearer picture of the human genome would particularly transform the treatment of multifactorial disorders such as breast and colorectal cancers, and Alzheimer's and Parkinson's diseases, where inherited risk has long been implicated but little understood. Genomics was expected to uncover the mechanisms of complex diseases, including asthma, hypertension, and diabetes. Vignettes were frequently proposed, featuring a patient visiting a doctor, who would order genetic testing that revealed certain genetic predispositions, allowing the doctor to craft a personalized approach to care, ensuring optimized prevention, diagnosis and treatment. There can be little doubt that these confident claims for genomic medicine were put forward in good faith. However, it was faith in an overly reductive and deterministic view of genetics, and in the ability of biomedical scientists and their clinical colleagues to translate the believed promise of genetic science into clinical reality. The gulf between genomics and personalized medicine turned out to be far greater than envisaged, resulting in an overstated optimism (Guttmacher & Collins, 2002; van Ommen et al., 1999) that, as mentioned, resulted in what now appear to have been quite unrealistic timescales (Collins, 1999).

It has emerged that even though markers of human variation (single nucleotide polymorphisms) can be associated with disease predisposition in large population samples, they contribute little to the apparent heritable risk and have poor predictive power at the individual level (Kraft & Hunter, 2009). Sequencing an individual's genome can produce a large amount of information, but the data is difficult to interpret, and so genomic medicine still has little effect on the health care of individuals (Collins, 2010; Hall et al., 2010).

The push to decode the genome carried with it an impetus to explore the ethical, legal and social implications of the new genetic knowledge, with the Human Genome Project dedicating five per cent of its budget to this cause. The program focused on clinical integration of genetic technology, public and professional education, and the fair use of genetic information, particularly in employment and health insurance (Collins, 1999). The aspiration to anticipate these implications before they transpire has been beneficial in allowing the formulation of appropriate guidelines and legislation, even though the timescales expected have proved awry (Ginsburg & Willard, 2009).

In terms of speculative ethics, therefore, genomic medicine stands as a beacon of hope. There has been speculation, some of which has been astray. Nevertheless, it has been limited in scope and concerted efforts have been made, and continue to be made, to tie in the scientific advances with considered ethical input and direction. The resulting liaison between the science and the ethics has been to the benefit of both.

3. Nanotechnology

The term "nanotechnology" was coined in 1974 by Norio Taniguchi (Taniguchi, 1974) and popularized in 1986 by Eric Drexler (who may have been unaware of its earlier usage) in his book "Engines of Creation: The Coming Era of Nanotechnology" (Drexler, 1986). "Nanotechnology" refers to the manipulation of matter at the atomic level. At this scale particles have different mechanical, electrical, thermal, optical and magnetic properties, possibly allowing the development of a whole range of materials and devices with new applications in fields as diverse as medicine and energy production. It has been postulated that nanomachines will one day be responsible for food production, biological repair, sewage processing, commodity fabrication, and house cleaning (Milburn, 2002).

Early discussions of molecular manufacturing were preoccupied with self-replicating nanomachines, and the prospect of the world being converted into a grey goo by these nanobots, a scenario sketched by Drexler in his seminal work (Drexler, 1986). Thus, a speculative doomsday scenario has characterized the field of nanotechnology from its earliest beginnings. Unfortunately, this has continued to dominate popular perception of nanotechnology (Sheetz et al., 2005), so much so that Drexler wishes he had never coined the term (Giles, 2004). He writes, "Fears associated with that old scenario are interfering with current research. . . . Researchers resent it and I want to clean up the mess." (Giles, 2004). Drexler now acknowledges that nanoscale manufacturing does not require self-replicating devices, and so this conjectural danger can be avoided through prohibition (Phoenix and Drexler, 2004). The most fruitful area of research to date has been the production of nanoscale particles, such as carbon nanotubes, for the manufacture of characteristic materials for use in electrical circuits, textiles, and cosmetics (Coyle et al., 2007; Mu & Sprando, 2010).

However, the fears provoked by the "grey goo" scenario have persisted, and apparently have been manipulated by some environmental groups to engender support for their present concerns regarding technology profiteering (Giles, 2004). By contrast, in informed circles the nanotechnology debate has settled down into less spectacular, but more substantive issues, such as the possible toxicity of nanomaterials (Xia et al., 2009), their effects on biological systems (Navarro et al., 2008) and the global economic effects of a possible nanotechnology revolution.

The relevance of this area for the present essay is the role of applied ethics in such ongoing debate. To what extent does bioethical commentary continue to grapple with speculative and alarmist scenarios? It is likely that the "grey goo" possibilities occupied attention that could otherwise have been directed towards the issues that ethicists are now focusing on, to far greater benefit. However, the dramatic and catastrophic threat described by Drexler's scenario seems to demand addressing. These typify the problems posed by speculative matters in applied ethics, which we will explore later.

4. Regenerative medicine

The term "regenerative medicine" first appeared in the literature in 1992 as a hypothetical future technology that could revolutionize clinical treatment (Kaiser, 1992). The idea gained momentum when embryonic stem cells were isolated in 1998 (Thomson et al., 1998), and the possible clinical significance of their growth potential and pluripotency was appreciated. In theory, damaged tissues and organs could be regenerated by insertion of stem cells, stimulation of endogenous stem cells, or transplantation of tissues or organs grown *in vitro* from the patient's own stem cells (Mironov et al., 2004). The underlying hope is that these techniques will radically advance the treatment of diseases as wide-ranging as Alzheimer's and Parkinson's diseases, diabetes and spinal cord injury.

As is often the case at the cutting edge of scientific development, exciting prospects raise unwarranted hopes bereft of a feasible scientific basis, and this has been particularly so in the field of regenerative medicine (Kirkpatrick et al., 2006). The prospects within regenerative medicine have captured the imagination of commentators from a variety of backgrounds, who too often have moved with undue haste from considering the use of stem cells to treat disease and disability to the potential to redesign human nature (Bostrom, 2005; Glannon, 2008; Ip, 2009b). Regenerative medicine is depicted by some as being "rich with Promethean promises"(Ip, 2009a, p. 3). It is here that we enter the realm of transhumanism and posthumanism, where ethicists have considered the implications of these in terms of the exacerbation of social inequalities, intergenerational fairness, environmental ethics, and the problems posed by endless life spans, with subsequent divergence of enhanced and unenhanced human species (Agar, 2007).

Far away from these highly speculative vistas, in today's laboratories the field of regenerative medicine faces complex difficulties that are hampering the clinical application of stem cells at the most basic level. For example, scientists are yet to ascertain how to reliably direct cell differentiation to the desired lineage and modify cells without raising the risk of tumor formation (Kirkpatrick et al., 2006). While this is a rapidly moving area of research, solutions to these basic problems will likely come gradually and hype should be tempered with caution (Daley, 2010).

Regenerative medicine raises bioethical challenges at different levels. Discussion that uncritically conflates regenerative medicine and its likely prospects with grandiose claims about remaking what it means to be human (e.g. Ip, 2009b) is profoundly misleading. Distaste over the latter claims may unfairly taint regenerative medicine, with the end-result of discouraging what could turn out to be extremely helpful medical interventions. While this may not be the intention of such commentators, it will only be avoided by clearly distinguishing the speculative hype from the serious science. Regenerative medicine in the clinic is not being driven by a program that views the human body as infinitely plastic, or that denies human finitude and mortality, and yet this is the concern of some who have been taken in by speculative hype (e.g. Song, 2009). Speculative bioethics of this ilk will simply perpetuate fundamental misconceptions.

Also of concern is the preoccupation of ethical debate on stem cells with the moral status of embryos. It is true that embryos are destroyed in the process of deriving embryonic stem cells. This is therefore a legitimate topic for debate and should not be avoided. However, this is not the sole area of bioethical debate on the potential of stem cells, especially as they relate to regenerative medicine. Lysaght and Campbell have cogently argued that bioethicists must also give due attention to the largely neglected issues of informed consent processes, the exploitation of women, the commodification of human tissue, science communication and the ownership of immortal cell lines (Lysaght & Campbell, 2011). All these are core ethical considerations for regenerative medicine as it seeks to enter the clinic. The fact that devoting attention to the issue of the embryo's moral status has left other important issues unattended shows the scarcity of moral consideration as a resource, and raises the question of how this consideration should be distributed. Speculative scenarios, with little if any relation to current clinical practice, such as the remaking of human nature through regenerative medicine, threaten to displace attention further from pressing current and emerging issues.

5. Cryonics

In simple terms cryonics is the practice of storing at very low temperatures the bodies or heads of legally deceased people (or animals), termed cryonic suspension. The purported value of cryonic suspension is that, from the stored body/head, the dead individual may be able to be resuscitated, allowing physical life after an indefinite period of death.

If there is a landmark publication for cryonics, it is Robert Ettinger's book "The Prospect of Immortality" (Ettinger, 1965). This is an attempt at a systematic evaluation of, and positive program for, the cryonics project. At the time of its publication no human bodies had been stored using cryonics, although the principle of freezing and reviving whole animals had been successfully demonstrated by Audrey Smith in the 1950s (Parry, 2004). Smith had succeeded in reviving some hamsters after freezing at -5 °C for 50-70 minutes, a minority of which survived for times approaching the normal hamster lifespan. However, Smith also established that this limited success disappeared if animals were frozen for longer than 70 minutes.

Presumably seeing the cup as half-full, Ettinger attempted to outline a viable approach to cryonics. Not a cryobiologist (he was a retired college maths and physics teacher at the time), Ettinger provided a semi-scientific evaluation of the problems facing the success of the cryonics enterprise, and an optimistic view of its eventual success. In a section entitled

"After a Moment of Sleep" (Ettinger, 1965, pp. 5-6) he describes a tired old man who will think of his death as merely a moment of dreamless sleep, like anaesthesia. This man will "awaken" unaware of the potentially vast period of time elapsed, and find himself in either a rejuvenated state, or about to undergo a process of "renovation". This can provide, if desired, the "physique of Charles Atlas". His "weary and faded wife" may also choose a physique to "rival Miss Universe" if she wishes. And, more importantly, "they will be gradually improved in mentality and personality". He imagines a future world which resembles "the present, king-sized and chocolate covered", in which "the resuscitees, will be not merely revived and cured, but enlarged and improved, made fit to work, play, and perhaps fight, on a grand scale and in a grand style." (Ettinger, 1965, p. 6)

With fanciful claims such as these in a foundational document of cryogenics, it is not surprising that the movement has been subject to ridicule. However, Ettinger acknowledges that "to remove the prospect of immortality from the realm of thin, hazy speculation or daydreams and secure it in the domain of emotional conviction and work-a-day policy... objections must be met, [and] a host of troublesome questions answered." (Ettinger, 1965, pp. 6-7) This is what his book aimed to do.

Many of the objections and troublesome questions may be of ethical importance. For instance, is cryonics impossible, perhaps even in principle? If so, are companies offering cryonic services being misleading at best or fraudulent at worst? What is the legal and moral status of the bodies in cryonic storage? If the claims of cryonicists are borne out in the future, what lives would the patients awake to, and could they reasonably be said to have consented to this given what they knew before they died? Should cryonics be judged more as a medical or mortuary procedure?

In order to evaluate cryonics ethically, it is necessary to know what the process might involve. In the light of this how likely is it that any of these currently impossible stages of the process will eventuate in the foreseeable future?

Cryonics may be divided into four stages: patient preparation and freezing, storage, renovation and resuscitation, and life. The first stage is the preparation and freezing of the cryonics patient. Here, the body of a patient is prepared for freezing, and rapidly cooled to a temperature below -120°C. Various procedures are undertaken by cryonicists with the aim of minimizing post-mortem damage to the body (see Best, 2008). This damage is in part what would occur to any body after breathing and blood circulation cease (broadly termed ischemic injury (Kerrigan & Stotland, 1993)), and in part injury that can result from the cooling process (mainly ice crystal formation (Best, 2008)).

Once the body is appropriately prepared, cooling to temperatures below -120°C occurs. The goal for cryonicists at this stage is to achieve vitreous cooling with the aim of avoiding the cellular damage caused by conventional freezing through ice crystal formation (Best, 2008). Cooling a large biological system like a human body to a contiguous vitreous state is not achievable at present – something cryonicists appear to freely admit (Fahy et al., 1990; Fahy, 2004). The main focus of cryonics is the resuscitation of the person who died (i.e. their identity or conscious self), not merely their body. Consequently, cryonics has tended to focus on achieving vitrification primarily in the part of the body they believe necessary for this to occur, *viz.*, the brain (Best, 2008), hoping that its smaller size will give greater chance of success. Many cryonics facilities offer storage for so-called "neuro-suspension or neuro-preservation" (Parry, 2004, p. 394) patients, namely, the preserved heads (with enclosed brain) of those who have died.

The second stage is the storage of the cooled cryonics patient at low temperatures until scientific advances make successful resuscitation possible. The main issue here seems to be storing the patient at a sufficiently low temperature that vitrification is maintained, yet high enough to minimize cracking and fracturing of the glassy, vitreous tissue which can occur at very low temperatures (Parry, 2004). A second issue in the storage phase is the maintenance of the patient in the cooled state continuously for an undefined period of time. This is dependent on the cryonic facilities being operational for that time, and also the storage being funded by the patient for the undefined duration - difficult matters to ensure with certainty.

The third stage is the renovation and resuscitation of the patient. Here speculation is at its most extreme. While there are considerable problems associated with the previous stages, these pale in comparison to the problems faced in thawing, repairing, reviving and perhaps enhancing the cryonics patient. However, cryonics has an in-built defence against these problems - the seemingly limitless potential for science and medicine to advance and overcome obstacles, if it is provided with sufficient time. The strength of cryonics is that the stored cryonics patients have plenty of time to spare.

Thus, while cryonicists give the impression of taking seriously the challenge of reducing obstacles to successful revival, there is always the possibility of appealing to speculative possibilities within future science as the solution. This means that scientific limitations do not have to be addressed too directly. Nevertheless, the potential problems are legion. These include: repair of whatever dysfunction or injury caused the death of the patient, and damage occurring between this time and freezing; repair of any damage caused by the first and second stages of cryonic intervention, such as toxic effects of the cryoprotectants, ice damage or fracturing of vitrified tissue; thawing the body, avoiding or treating de-vitrification (cellular collapse) and any other damage caused; removal of cryoprotectants and reperfusion of the body with blood, while avoiding reperfusion-induced injury; any problems associated with reviving the conscious person from their deceased state, to a healthy and possibly enhanced state.

Cryonicists argue that these seem like huge problems from the point of view of current science and technology. A strong theme underlying their confidence in the power of future science and technology is often a highly reductive view of biology and medicine. According to this, all of the problems mentioned above are simply a matter of atoms being in the wrong configuration within a biological system; move the atoms into the correct configuration and energy state, and the patient is resuscitated. The clearest statement of this is provided by Merkle (1992, pp. 6-7): "... the purpose of medicine is to change arrangements of atoms that are 'unhealthy' to arrangements of atoms that are 'healthy'."

From this reductive view, future developments in medicine will involve gaining better control over our ability to manipulate atoms - medicine (especially that involved in cryonics) will be a matter of nanotechnology (Merkle, 1992). The cryonics community's endorsement of nanotechnology is probably not welcome news to those scientists studying the behaviour of matter on a very small scale. In fact nanoscientists have often sought to distance themselves from this type of science fiction speculation (Milburn, 2002) in much the same way as cryobiologists have sought to distance themselves from cryonics.

The speculation increases even further when considering the life awaiting a resuscitated cryonics patient. An idealistic vision is exemplified by Ettinger's claim that "You and I, as resuscitees, may awaken still old, but before long we will gambol with the spring lambs - not to mention the young chicks, our wives." (Ettinger, 1965, p. 63). Less optimistic, but equally speculative, possibilities could include life in an impaired mental or physical state as a result of imperfect techniques - a life with unforeseen suffering, perhaps that one might judge not worth living. Another might be that continuity of consciousness is lost, causing the revived person to effectively be a new individual without any memory of their previous pre-resuscitation life (that such loss may occur is even admitted by a cryonicist (Best, 2008)).

5.1 What is an appropriate ethical analysis of cyronics?

Each of the stages of cryonics as it is currently practised and envisioned by cryonicists is a potential focus of ethical scrutiny. Cryonics is regarded by its adherents as an indefinitely prolonged medical procedure. Considering it from this point of view, it should be analyzed as such, opening up a vast array of medical ethical considerations. For example, is the consent given by the cryonics patient adequate considering the unknown nature of much of what the full procedure may entail? Should patients be able to undergo cryonic preservation before legal death, when cryonicists claim it would be more likely to be effective? A practical legal issue is the property status of the revived person and their body. As current law stands in most jurisdictions in which cryonicists operate, property rights over the deceased person's body are ceded to the cryonics company (it is treated as a bequeathed cadaver) - is this reversible if the cadaver comes back to life? What is the moral and legal status of the frozen body, and what implications does this have for the standard of care provided by the cryonics facility? Is the prolonging of individual lives (potentially indefinitely, according to cryonicists' vision of future medicine) morally wrong, justifiable, or perhaps even required? And if the latter, should public funding be provided for the practice and for research to further its development and use?

Alternatively, cryonics could be viewed as an intricate and expensive mortuary procedure. From this point of view a largely different analysis emerges, characterized by different issues. For example, since cryonics is not marketed as an alternative to embalming and burial or cremation, are people who enter the contract being defrauded? What should be made of the (on this account) mistaken beliefs of those practising and undertaking the procedure? Should the wishes of cryonics patients be respected posthumously, especially when these are wishes that can (or, at best, may) never be realized? Is cryonics a repugnant use of a dead body, and, if so, does this have any normative implications?

Depending on one's judgment of the future success of cryonics, two quite different, and ultimately incompatible, avenues of ethical consideration will be pursued. It should be noted that, for those stored cryonically and for cryonicists, the decision of whether cryonics should be treated more or less speculatively by bioethicists is nothing less than a matter of life or death. Cryonics patients are at risk by their being incorrectly treated as cadavers - for example undermining research into their reanimation, and giving insufficient support for their care while in storage. The quality of their future lives is also at risk through insufficient preparation for eventual reanimation. Should bioethicists consider these questions even though they may be skeptical about the science? If the claims and objectives of cryonics are taken seriously, to focus on the wrong question could be decried as being complicit in killing (or perhaps letting die), or at best harming, these patients (Nordmann, 2007).

How should ethicists decide between these two possibilities? One option is to consider both, however this means that a great deal of time is devoted to considering highly speculative possibilities, which may never eventuate. Perhaps the likelihood of one or the other being correct should be estimated, and the lower probability, speculative scenario eschewed in favour of the other. This grounds ethical analysis in reasonable scientific understanding and expectation, and confines ethics to those moral issues that are currently present—in this case, the current reality of individuals having their cadavers frozen and stored indefinitely postmortem—rather than those that may never exist at all.

6. The problems of speculation in ethics

It is worth remembering what may be at stake, both in the case of cryonics, but also for speculative matters more broadly. If considerable attention is devoted to speculative possibilities like cryonics, what is at stake is the neglect of more current moral issues from which practical and ethical attention has, to some degree, been diverted (Nordmann, 2007). Whatever response one might make will have to take note of competing priorities: to devote attention to the ethical demands made by suffering due to famine, environmental disasters, or war, the needs of the infertile, the chronically sick or the terminally ill, against the demands of those who have freely decided to undergo cryonics in the hope of a better life at some indefinite time in an indefinite future.

One problem of speculative ethics is epistemological - the more speculative and removed from present experience possibilities become, the more uncertain our knowledge becomes. It will have little in common with current technology. For example, Drexler's speculative ideas about self-replicating nanomachines bore little resemblance to nanotechnology at the time he published *Machines of Creation*. Moreover, it bears little resemblance to current nanotechnology, which has advanced significantly in the manufacturing of nanoscale products using techniques such as self-assembly, rather than the more fanciful nano-machines of Drexler's speculation. While Drexler's general idea of the way in which nanotechnology will develop is not necessarily false (only time can determine this), there is little relationship between these speculative visions and existing technologies. This may do intense disservice to existing technologies and the way in which they are perceived (Jones, 2006).

However, like all empirical predictions about the way a technology will emerge or develop, speculations, such as those of Drexler, may indeed be false. In this way, speculative claims informing ethical reasoning suffer from the same weakness that afflicts the empirical version of slippery slope arguments. Empirical slippery slope arguments rest on an empirical prediction, arguing that (acceptable) policy or situation A will, as a result of social or psychological tendencies, result in the emergence of (unacceptable) policy or situation B. Like any forward-looking empirical claim, it is open to challenges on its assumptions about social or psychological tendencies or whatever mechanism is being used to justify the claim.

An overarching problem is that it is usually only in retrospect that we can know with any certainty whether our speculations or prognostications were accurate. Also of relevance to this discussion is our inability to predict future scientific developments with reliable accuracy. One only has to think of once assured dicta that, with hindsight, proved unwarranted obstacles to further research. There was the alleged inability of the central nervous system to regenerate to any discernible extent after birth, or to replace any of its neurons (Ramon y Cajal, 1928). Alongside this can be placed the alleged impossibility of cloning in mammals (McGrath & Solter, 1984). We have already discussed the opposite phenomenon, which is the occurrence of obstacles that either were not predicted, or were underestimated. Clearly, when dealing with predictions, ethicists, as much as other philosophers, scientists, and policy makers, need to be wary.

A second problem is that these epistemological problems have moral consequences. As ethics becomes more speculative, its relation to the technology that it is discussing grows increasingly tenuous. This raises problems we have already touched on. First, it diverts ethical attention away from current concerns pertaining to the technology, concerns often in need of ethical attention. Second, the speculative moral judgments about a technology can influence current perceptions of it. Hence, an emerging technology can be smothered or hampered, either by the weight of enthusiastic speculative expectations (such as has arguably been the case for genomic medicine (Evans et al., 2011)), or by the weight of moral and social condemnation as a result of the harmful implications of the speculative aspects of the technology (such as the grey goo scenario for nanotechnology). Both can have unjustly negative consequences for the technology under discussion.

Applied ethics must be applicable to some ethical issue or problem. Unfortunately, speculative ethics relates to speculative. Consider the ethical discussion on genetic testing in assisted reproductive technologies (ARTs) regarding whether embryos with particular genetic combinations should or should not be implanted in a woman for further development. While a much of this work has addressed pressing issues such as the moral status of these types of procedures and the implications this may have for social regulation of reproductive choices, a troublingly large portion of this work anticipates or presupposes a future in which the desired genetic composition of a child can be determined or when all human reproduction is handled by technological means such as these (Sharma, 2007; Steinbock, 2008). Excessive concentration on the latter at the expense of the former is paying more attention to speculative scenarios far removed from current scientific reality than to current applied ethical considerations. Speculative ethics does not conform to paradigmatic work in applied ethics, in that it addresses imaginary (and perhaps never to be realized) moral problems, not extant, or often even very likely, practical problems.

This raises the question of whether ethicists should be free to consider whatever they like, or as we are arguing, should their attention be directed towards particular issues and projects? Moral reflection is not an infinite resource and this leads to the question of how it should best be distributed. One plausible way of distributing a scarce resource is to do so in a way that maximizes benefit. The *prima facie* case described here is that, unlike paradigmatic applied ethics, the benefits of speculative ethics are not clear, since it does not directly address extant moral problems (Nordmann, 2007; Nordmann & Rip, 2009).

We argue that, since those engaging in speculative ethics are doing so *at the expense* of addressing real (i.e. not imaginary) moral issues, there is a distributive justice problem here. This allows ongoing moral problems to persist, whether these be problems related to famine, harmful exploitation of the vulnerable, or health inequalities. These wrongs and the suffering they cause are immense and are currently occurring. The obligation to use moral reflection to address these problems ought to be a concern for every moral philosopher, motivating them to seek as just a distribution of their discipline's work as possible. If these problems and many like them are taken seriously, they lead to a commitment to work on problems like these rather than on highly speculative ones.

Thus, speculative ethics may squander the benefit that can be derived from the application of moral reasoning to current problems. However, speculative ethics may go further than this, reducing the potential of some current and emerging technologies to realize their benefits for society, and in this way diminishing the means available for addressing current problems. Examples already alluded to include nanotechnology and the self-replicating nanobots and "grey goo" scenarios, and regenerative medicine with speculative concerns about radical life extension and a posthuman future.

A related manner in which speculative ethics can negatively affect current and emerging technology is the flipside of the first. This technology can be overwhelmed by a weight of expectation that it is unable to match. This has arguably been the case for genomic technologies, with their expectation of ushering in a new era of personalized medicine with its tailored pharmacological and behavioural prevention and treatment of disease (Collins, 1999).

This raises an interesting issue since in this case the problems have been created more by scientists than by ethicists. Much of the hype has come from scientists within the field, perhaps "talking up" the potential impact of their work in an attempt to gain research grants in an extremely competitive funding market, and also reflecting excitement at the promise certain emerging technologies might hold (Evans et al., 2011). As outlined earlier, the director of the National Human Genome Research Institute in 1999 anticipated the hugely beneficial effect that genomics would have on medicine by 2010 (Collins, 1999). Collins does caution that his vision has obstacles to its realization, but the ones he identifies are not scientific, but rather ethical and practical. According to Collins (1999) ethical and regulatory hurdles must urgently be addressed to ensure that genetic information is not misused, and health professionals, such as medical genetic specialists, must be educated to ensure that they are up to the task of understanding and treating patients using genomic medicine.

The moral imperative that Collins asserts is an example of what Nordmann has referred to as "foreshortening of the conditional", a general problem that he claims underlies much speculative ethics (Nordmann, 2007; Nordmann and Rip, 2009). He characterizes such speculative moral claims as having the conditional form: if conditions C obtain, then speculative scenario A will occur, and this will create or exacerbate ethical issues I^1, I^2, and so forth. The foreshortening of this conditional statement occurs when the "if" becomes subsumed by the "then", which he claims creates a mandate for action with respect to the scenario and the ethical issues that arise:

> 'If-and-then' statements begin by suggesting possible technological developments and then indicate consequences that seem to demand immediate attention. What looks like a merely possible, and definitely speculative future in the first half of the sentence (the 'if'), turns into something inevitable in the second half (the 'then'). As the hypothetical gets displaced by a supposed actual, the imagined future overwhelms the present (Nordmann & Rip, 2009, p. 273).

Thus:

> The true and perfectly legitimate conditional "if we ever were in the position to conquer the natural ageing process and become immortal, then we would face the question whether withholding immortality is tantamount to murder" becomes foreshortened to "if you call into question that biomedical research can bring about immortality within some relevant period of time, you are complicit with murder" – no matter how remote the possibility that such research might succeed, we are morally obliged to support it (Nordmann, 2007, p. 33).

Collins' speculative vision of personalized genomic medicine in 2010 was false. As a result of highly optimistic predictions such as this and others (Epstein, 2004), many of the promises of genomic medicine remain unfulfilled (Evans et al., 2011) despite considerable progress being made. It is now being asked whether time and money spent on genomic medicine has been wasted, or would have been better spent elsewhere, such as on population-based public health strategies to reduce smoking, obesity and risky alcohol use (Hall et al., 2010; Holtzman & Marteau, 2000). Nordmann (2009) argues that dramatic promises such as these are often made with regard to emerging technologies, and they support the "conditional foreshortening" arguments that he maintains provide much of the impetus for speculative ethics.

Evans et al. (2011) argue that conjectures, like that of Collins, about future developments within science and technology can be – perhaps counter-intuitively – an impediment to their development. This is because they can underestimate the number and extent of hurdles that must be overcome in the course of development, and overestimate the benefits of their particular approach as a means to address problems. The combination of these factors means that other potentially promising approaches can be overlooked, leading to a crippling misallocation of resources, which can endanger the sustainability of the field (Evans et al., 2011). In addition, scientific and technological promises made are frequently not delivered on, which undermines the legitimacy of science in general, and the field from which the speculation arises in particular (Nordmann & Rip, 2009). This helps to explain the distance that many scientists seek from hyperbolic interpretations of their work (such as those working within nanotechnology and cryogenic science). A realistic appraisal of current and future developments in science, and the promises made about science and technological development, is needed in order for it to receive the level of trust and support that it deserves, but also, and perhaps more importantly, to allow for the allocation of research resources to those areas of most (genuine) promise and moral relevance.

Applying this approach to cryonics draws attention to the number and enormity of the scientific hurdles that must be overcome in order for reanimation of stored bodies to be possible, assuming that this is possible, even in principle. However, as mentioned above, the peculiar nature of cryonics affords its devotees a response to objections of this kind, namely, that the bodies can be maintained in storage until such time as science has developed techniques for repairing and reviving them. Thus the fact that time-consuming scientific hurdles must be overcome is not *in itself* seen as a problem with respect to the revival of the stored bodies. However, the longer it takes for these hurdles to be overcome, the more likely it is that other factors will arise to thwart or displace cryogenic aims, such as the possibility that medical advances will extend human life to the extent that cryonics becomes irrelevant. However, this assumes that revival of cryonically stored bodies is possible, *and* that continuity of strong personal psychological identity is maintained in the revived body – both extremely dubious assumptions.

While cryonics is an extreme illustration of speculation, both scientific and ethical, it typifies the problems of speculative ethics. The example of Collins shows that even relatively modest speculation can be problematic. These problems amount to a strong case for the rejection of speculative ethics in favour of grounding ethics in realistic and rigorous appraisals of science and technology, and a focus on current and imminent concerns.

7. Exploring Roache's defence of speculation

Our evaluation of speculative ethics would be incomplete without looking seriously at a counter analysis in its favour. Roache's (2008) article aims to defend speculative ethics against the objections we have so far leveled at it, so it is important we explore it here. Roache begins by pointing out the important role of thought experiments in philosophy, which are highly imaginative and serve to test and analyze our intuitions, while noting that these are imaginative analytic tools, rather than speculations about possible future events. Also, she argues that a vast amount of ethical thinking involves anticipating, evaluating, and choosing among possible future events – often very mundane ones – many of which will not come to pass.

Roache's main argument can be summed up like this. (1) Some speculative future possibilities may be great potential harms or goods. (2) We ought to determine which speculative future possibilities are harmful or beneficial, so that the former can be avoided and the latter pursued; ethical analysis is required to make these value judgments. Therefore, (3) we ought to give ethical consideration to future possibilities.

This allows ethics to be in the business not merely of considering and solving current and emerging problems, but also of shaping the direction of social and scientific development away from future harms or towards future goods. To do otherwise would be to let science and society develop without any moral guidance, allowing ethicists only the job of solving problems once they have arisen or are imminent. She argues that many of our most important projects are the result of moral evaluation of a problem and speculation about potential future solutions to it. She cites as examples the development of the ARTs that allow the selective implantation of embryos, as a response to the moral problem of genetic disorders, and carbon capture technology as a response to the problem of global warming. In one respect, these examples do not serve her position well. They are both examples of current, not speculative, moral problems, for which technological responses are developed. Devoting the scarce resource of moral attention to these is therefore acceptable to the anti-speculation position. However, the development of solutions to these moral problems may require speculation about the nature of possible solutions, and the evaluation of these to determine which ones ought to be pursued. Roache argues that, without this moral engagement with speculative possibilities, scientific resources may be squandered by pursuing solutions that are morally problematic, or not maximally beneficial.

A difficulty with Roache's main argument arises with the quantifiers. Premise one can be accepted. However, even if we accept that *some* speculative and unlikely possibilities are worthy of ethical consideration, we must still determine which possibilities these are. This requires that all possible future possibilities must be imagined and ethically evaluated, no matter how unlikely. Thus the correct conclusion to the above argument is that we ought to give ethical consideration to *all* future possibilities. Given the consideration that ethicists are a scarce resource, it makes sense that their time should be spent wisely. Among the infinitely many speculative possibilities, and the vast number of actualities to which ethicists could direct their attention, it is plausible to argue that it would be best for them to attend to those that are most significant morally and most likely to eventuate. She disagrees, arguing that even moves to restrict scope to only those possibilities that are not known to be highly unlikely are misguided. She cites two counter examples, and she uses these as evidence that we take seriously highly unlikely possibilities when they promise great harm or benefit. First is the possibility that the Large Hadron Collider will create a black hole that will destroy the earth, which was the basis for a lawsuit to halt its activity (Boyle, 2008); second is the fact that heroic efforts are often expended to provide benefit (such as attempting to save a life) even when this is the least likely outcome.

The example of the Large Hadron Collider lawsuit is question-begging. While it does show that the plaintiffs took seriously the threat that they believed the Large Hadron Collider could pose to the future of the world, it does not show that anyone else did, or, more importantly, that anyone would be *right* to. The argument mounted by the plaintiffs is arguably an example of what Stich (1978) calls a "Doomsday Argument". This is an argument based on the principle that prohibition is required of any activity that holds a non-zero chance of causing an unthinkably immense catastrophe. Such a principle would prohibit a vast amount of innocuous work (in the sciences and elsewhere). For example, there may be a non-zero possibility that a chemical synthesized in a laboratory may initiate a chain-reaction that obliterates the ozone layer, destroying all life on earth. However, prohibiting all chemical synthesis based on this possibility would be ridiculous. Van der Burg notes that these "Doomsday Arguments" are a philosophically uninteresting variant of slippery slope arguments, in which the objected-to outcome "is so highly speculative that the cogency of the argument—insofar as it exists—depends more upon the horror than upon the likelihood [of it occurring]" (van der Burg, 1991, p. 43).

More challenging is Roache's example of heroic attempts to save a life, such as a child trapped in a cave. A search and rescue team is available; however, it is highly unlikely that they will find the child alive. We may, she contends, react with horror to the suggestion that, in light of the small probability of success, it is not worth the cost (in terms of time, resources, risk of injury) deploying the search and rescue team. She argues that the value of the child's life is such that we deem it worth these heroic efforts, despite their highly unlikely chance of success.

Clearly we *do* undertake these, but, as with the previous example, this does not show that we are always right to do so, nor does it show why we might be right to. It is worth noting that, if the rescue is undertaken, it may not be justified by the value of the speculative outcome, but by the consequences of the undertaking *regardless of outcome*. For example, in this case, the institution of child-rearing may be negatively affected by parents believing that the state will abandon their children in times of great need, hence the rescue must proceed. At an abstract level, the resources expended in such an endeavour may produce greater benefit if spent elsewhere, say improving public health in third-world countries, or providing vaccinations. However, Roache's example is a practical one, and the rescue team cannot be deployed to third-world countries to work on sanitation systems there. In other words, this example is disanalogous in terms of deciding which speculative possibilities are worth taking seriously in applied ethics and pursuing as a society. Nevertheless, we might adjust the scenario to minimize this problem, by having other children lost in other caves within the rescuer's area. Differences in the nature of the caves and the children make the chances of success finding some more likely than others. There are enough rescuers to undertake some of the rescues immediately, while others must wait. In this situation it is reasonable to undertake those rescues with the greatest chance of success, or at least not to undertake those *known to be highly unlikely* while others wait.

In light of these considerations, Roache's example fails to show that we are wrong to eschew options known to be highly unlikely in favour of other more likely options. But the example does show that highly improbable, but highly valuable possibilities, may still make moral demands on us. However, these are demands that must be weighed among the many demands of other social, scientific and technological options. Roache acknowledges that some projects will be unacceptably speculative and, given resource constraints, more worthwhile options should be pursued in their stead. One could, therefore, think that she endorses the kind of weighting that favours options addressing current or imminent concerns over those that are distant and speculative (other things being equal).

Nevertheless, she argues against this focus on "socially beneficial" outcomes, the judgment of which she says is highly fallible, and influenced by factors such as fads, prejudice, bias, and misconception. We would, therefore, have reason to view such a focus as being shortsighted and misguided. To illustrate this point she uses the example of bacterial antibiotic resistance, which she rightly states could render all antibiotics ineffective against bacterial infection. She argues that this is not a current problem, since there are still drugs that can treat the relevant diseases. She is right that there are drugs or drug combinations that can be effective in treating antibiotic resistant diseases. She is also correct in asserting that the emergence of bacterial strains that are resistant to *all* antibiotics and their combinations is not a current problem, and therefore could be excluded from a moral focus that privileges current over future problems. However, she is wrong to infer that antibiotic resistance *per se* is not a current problem, and this undermines her example.

A brief examination of *Staphlococcus aureus* is sufficient to reveal this. Penicillin resistant *S. aureus* was a significant comorbidity during the influenza pandemic of 1957 and 1958 (Kunin, 1993; Schoenbaum, 2001), and, more recently, Methicillin-resistant *S. aureus* (MRSA) was reported to increase mortality during the 2003-2004 and 2006-2007 influenza seasons by 33 per cent. Meta-analysis of 31 articles published from 1980-2000 revealed that patients with MRSA infection have significantly greater odds of mortality compared to otherwise similar patients with Methicillin-susceptible *S. aureus* (Cosgrove et al., 2003), despite the fact that at the time, MRSA was uniformly susceptible to treatment with Vancomycin (which is no longer the case (Hiramatsu, 2001)). *S. Aureus* is one of many such bacteria that exhibit rapid development of antibiotic resistance and pose a current problem to successful treatment. Collectively, these findings show that her example fails as an example of a merely future problem. The future development of alternatives to antibiotics is an approach that would be effective for this current problem *as well* as solving the future problem of total antibiotic resistance in pathogenic bacteria. Her example shows that—contrary to her own argument— an emphasis on current or imminent problems can yield solutions that are not shortsighted, but beneficial now and in the probable future.

However, the point Roache is making is that there are serious future problems that we are right to anticipate and devote our efforts towards solving. Although there would be benefits to a cheap alternative to antibiotics now, even if this were not the case, we would be right to devote resources to considering the moral implications of total antibiotic resistance, and making efforts to develop alternatives to antibiotic use. Roache is correct in stating that a position committing one only to considering current and imminent problems may fail to prepare for or avoid some harmful future scenarios. It may also fail to identify beneficial or harmful future scenarios. Despite their improbability, they may still be significant enough to be worth our current attention. However, given the highly contingent nature of many speculative possibilities, a *prima facie* preference towards consideration of current and imminent problems seems reasonable. Roache's arguments against this restriction of scope are only partially successful; she does not challenge the value of current moral problems and she acknowledges that many speculative possibilities are so unlikely that attending to them would be a waste of time (Roache, 2008). We are then left in the middle ground of admitting a legitimate place for speculative possibilities in moral thinking, but requiring that these be weighed against actual or imminent issues.

How we weigh up the many current and potential future issues that could be attended to is a difficult question. We suggest that relevant factors include a realistic and scientifically rigorous assessment of the harms and benefits that each issue contains, *and* the likelihood that future aspects might be realized. Roache makes the suggestion that "Reflecting on where our most important values lie, and how we might work to maximise them, is surely an important step towards ensuring that ethical concern, and other valuable resources, are not squandered" (Roache, 2008, p. 326). This is a good suggestion, which is compatible with the middle-ground arrived at here. It should be noted that multiple values would also have to be balanced against each other, thus prioritizing is inevitable.

Applying this to cryonics, we may decide, upon careful reflection, that one of our most important values entails sustaining individual lives through the pursuit of life-extending technologies such as this. In that case, full-blown cryonics is a live ethical issue, and we should seriously consider taking steps to realize its potential. However, the highly speculative nature of cryonics means that we can only have limited confidence that it is a good means of pursuing that which we value. Moreover, a value that entails life-prolonging technologies such as this would likely entail the promotion of life-prolonging possibilities elsewhere. Maximization of this value would arguably require a much greater focus on more reliable or likely means for prolonging life, such as public health measures in third-world countries. Revisiting our modification of Roache's analogy of rescuing the trapped child may be useful here. In cryonics, there may be a possibility that the frozen cryonics patients can be 'rescued' by future medicine. However, this is a rescue effort of highly unlikely success, whereas there are other efforts in which success is vastly more likely. To pursue the unlikely alternative at the expense of those that are so vastly more likely would amount to irresponsible allocation of resources.

8. Conclusion

The degree to which ethics as a discipline should engage with highly speculative possibilities is a significant matter at a time when science fact and fiction are becoming increasingly difficult to disentangle (Jones, 2006). Cryonics has been used as a paradigmatic example, the extreme nature of which highlights the issues involved for bioethicists. We have argued that considerable caution is required when approaching all speculative situations; the more extreme the situation the more cautious the response should be. Even if it is conceded that speculation can be a useful tool for ethical reasoning, and that the pursuit of speculative possibilities may in principle be justifiable, it is far from clear that the highly speculative, like cryonics, offers sufficient likelihood of benefit to warrant consideration, let alone prioritization ahead of more likely and beneficial future possibilities. Tempting as it may be for bioethicists to be swept away by the apparently exciting and enticing possibilities rampant in the literature, moves in the direction of speculative ethics ought to be made with extreme caution.

9. References

Agar, N. (2007). Whereto Transhumanism? The Literature Reaches a Critical Mass. *Hastings Center Report,* Vol. 37, No. 3, (May-June 2007), pp. 12-7, eISSN 1552 -146X, ISSN 0093 0334.

Bailey, R. (2005). *Liberation Biology: The Scientific and Moral Case for the Biotech Revolution,* Prometheus Books, Amherst, ISBN-10: 159-1022274, ISBN-13: 978-1591022275, NY.

Best, B. P. (2008). Scientific Justification of Cryonics Practice. *Rejuvenation Research,* Vol. 11, No. 2, pp. 493-503.

Bostrom, N. (2005). A History of Transhumanist Thought. *Journal of Evolution and Technology,* Vol. 14, No. 1, (April 2005), pp. 1-25, ISSN 1541- 0099.

Boyle, A. (2008), 'Doomsday Fears Spark Lawsuit over Collider'. In: *MSNBC,* April 4 2011, Retrieved from: <http://www.msnbc.msn.com/id/23844529/ns/technology_and_science-science/>.

Collins, F. (1999). Medical and Societal Consequences of the Human Genome Project. *New England Journal of Medicine,* Vol. 341, No. 1, (July 1999), pp. 28-37 ISSN 0028-4793, eISSN 1533-4406.

Collins, F. (2010). Has the Revolution Arrived? *Nature,* Vol. 464, No. 7289, (April, 2010), pp. 674- 675, eISSN 1476 - 4687.

Cosgrove, S. E., et al. (2003). Comparison of Mortality Associated with Methicillin-Resistant and Methicillin-Susceptible Staphylococcus Aureus Bacteremia: A Meta-Analysis. *Clinical Infectious Diseases,* Vol. 36, pp. 53-59, eISSN 1537-6591, ISSN 1058-4838.

Coyle, S., et al. (2007). Smart Nanotextiles: A Review of Materials and Applications. *MRS Bulletin,* Vol. 32, No. 5, (May 2007), pp. 434-42.

Daley, G. Q. (2010). Stem Cells: Roadmap to the Clinic. *The Journal of Clinical Investigation,* Vol. 120, No. 1, (January, 2010), pp. 8-10, ISSN 0021-9738, eISSN1558-8238.

Drexler, K. E. (1986). Engines of Creation, Anchor / DoubleDay, ISBN 0-385-19972-4, New York

Epstein, C. J. (2004). Genetic Testing: Hope or Hype? Genetics in Medicine, Vol. 6, No. 4, pp. 165-72

Ettinger, R. (1965). *The Prospect of Immortality,* Sidgwick and Johnson, Retrieved from <http://www.cryonics.org/book1.html>

Evans, J. P., Meslin, E. M., Marteau, T. M., & Caulfield, T. (2011). Deflating the Genomic Bubble. *Science,* Vol. 331, No. 6019, (February, 2011), pp. 861-2, eISSN 1095 -9203.

Fahy, G. (2004). Cryopreservation of Organs by Vitrification: Perspectives and Recent Advances. *Cryobiology,* Vol. 48, No. 2, (April 2004), pp. 157-78, ISSN 0011-2240.

Fahy, G., Saur, J., & Williams, R. J. (1990). Physical Problems with the Vitrification of Large Biological Systems. Cryobiology, Vol. 27, (October 1990), pp. 492-510, ISSN 0011-2240.

Garreau, J. (2005), 'Let Humanity Prevail', *The Age,* August 11.

Giles, J. (2004). Nanotech Takes Small Step Towards Burying 'Grey Goo'. *Nature,* Vol. 429, No. 6992, (June 2004), pp. 591, eISSN 1476-4687.

Ginsburg, G. S. & Willard, H. F. (2009). Genomic and Personalized Medicine: Foundations and Applications. Translational Research: The Journal of Laboratory and Clinical Medicine, Vol. 154, No. 6, (December 2009), pp. 277-87, ISSN 1931-5244, ISSN 0022-2143.

Glannon, W. (2008). Decelerating and Arresting Human Aging, In: *Medical Enhancement and Posthumanity,* B. Gordijn and R. Chadwick, pp. 175-89, Springer, ISBN 978-1-4020-8851-3, Dordrecht; London.

Guttmacher, A. E. & Collins, F. S. (2002). Genomic Medicine--a Primer. *The New England Journal of Medicine,* Vol. 347, No. 19, (November 2002), pp. 1512-20, ISSN 0028-4793, eISSN 1533-4406.

Habermas, J. (2003). The Future of Human Nature, Polity Press, ISBN 0-7456-2986-5, Cambridge.

Hall, W. D., Mathews, R., & Morley, K. I. (2010). Being More Realistic About the Public Health Impact of Genomic Medicine. *PLoS Medicine,* Vol. 7, No. 10,(October 2010), p. e1000347, ISSN 1549-1277, eISSN 1549-1676.

Hiramatsu, K. (2001). Vancomycin-Resistant Staphylococcus Aureus: A New Model of Antibiotic Resistance. *The Lancet Infectious Diseases,* Vol. 1, No.3, (October 2001), pp. 147-55, ISSN 1473-3099.

Holtzman, N. A. & Marteau, T. M. (2000). Will Genetics Revolutionize Medicine? *New England Journal of Medicine,* Vol. 343, No. 2, (July, 2000), pp. 141-44, ISSN 0028-4793, eISSN 1533-4406.

Ip, K.-T. (2009a). Introduction: Regenerative Medicine at the Heart of the Culture Wars, In: *The Bioethics of Regenerative Medicine,* K.-T. Ip, pp. 3-10, Springer, ISBN 978-1-4020-8966-4, Netherlands.

Ip, K.-T. (Ed.). (2009b). *The Bioethics of Regenerative Medicine*, Springer, ISBN 978-1-4020-8966-4, Netherlands.

Jones, D. G. (2006). Enhancement: Are Ethicists Excessively Influenced by Baseless Speculations? *Medical Humanities,* Vol. 32, No. 2, (September 2006), pp. 77-81.

Kaiser, L. R. (1992). The Future of Multihospital Systems. *Topics in Health Care Financing,* Vol. 18, No. 4, pp. 32-45.

Kerrigan, C. L. & Stotland, M. A. (1993). Ischemia Reperfusion Injury: A Review. *Microsurgery,* Vol. 14, No. 3, (October 1993), pp. 165-75, eISSN 1098-2752.

Kirkpatrick, C. J., et al. (2006). Visions for Regenerative Medicine: Interface between Scientific Fact and Science Fiction. *Artificial Organs,* Vol. 30, No. 10, (October, 2006), pp. 822-7, ISSN 1525-1594.

Kraft, P. & Hunter, D. J. (2009). Genetic Risk Prediction - Are We There Yet? *The New England Journal of Medicine,* Vol. 360, No. 17, (April 2009), pp. 1701-3, ISSN 0028-4793, eISSN 1533-4406.

Kunin, C. M. (1993). Resistance to Antimicrobial Drugs - a Worldwide Calamity. *Annals of Internal Medicine,* Vol. 118, No.7, (April 1993), pp. 557-61, ISSN 0003-4819.

Lysaght, T. & Campbell, A. V. (2011). The Ethics of Regenerative Medicine: Broadening the Scope Beyond the Moral Status of Embryos, *Third GABEX International Meeting,* Tokyo, February 2001.

McGrath, J., & Solter, D. (1984). Inability of Mouse Blastomere Nuclei Transferred to Enucleated Zygotes to Support Development in Vitro. *Science,* Vol. 226, No. 4680, (December 1984), pp. 1317-9, ISNN 0036-8075.

Merkle, R. C. (1992). The Technical Feasibility of Cryonics. Medical Hypotheses, Vol. 39, pp. 6-16

Milburn, C. (2002). Nanotechnology in the Age of Posthuman Engineering: Science Fiction as Science. *Configurations,* Vol. 10, No.2 (Spring 2002),pp. 261-95, eISSN 1080-6520, ISSN 1063-1801.

Mironov, V., Visconti, R. P., & Markwald, R. R. (2004). What Is Regenerative Medicine? Emergence of Applied Stem Cell and Developmental Biology. *Expert Opinion on Biological Therapy,* Vol. 4, No. 6, (June 2004), pp. 773-81, ISSN 1471-2598, eISSN 1744-7682.

Mu, L. & Sprando, R. L. (2010). Application of Nanotechnology in Cosmetics. *Pharmaceutical Research,* Vol.27, No.8,(August 2010), pp. 1-4, ISSN 0724-8741, eISSN 1573-904X.

Navarro, E., et al. (2008). Environmental Behavior and Ecotoxicity of Engineered Nanoparticles to Algae, Plants, and Fungi. *Ecotoxicology,* Vol. 17, No. 5, (July 2008), pp. 372-86, ISSN 0963-9292, eISSN 1573-3017.

Nordmann, A. (2007). If and Then: A Critique of Speculative Nanoethics. *NanoEthics,* Vol. 1, pp. 31-46

Nordmann, A. & Rip, A. (2009). Mind the Gap Revisited. *Nature Nanotechnology,* Vol. 4, No. 5, pp. 273-74

Parry, B. (2004). Technologies of Immortality: The Brain on Ice. *Studies in the History and Philosophy of Biology & Biomedical Science,* Vol. 35, No. 2, (June 2004), pp. 391-413, ISSN 1369-8486.

Phoenix, C. & Drexler, E. (2004). Safe Exponential Manufacturing. *Nanotechnology,* Vol. 15, No. 8, (august, 2004),pp. 869-72, ISSN 0957-4484, eISSN 1361- 6528.

Ramon y Cajal, S. (1928). Degeneration and Regeneration of the Nervous System, Hafner, New York.

Roache, R. (2008). Ethics, Speculation, and Values. *NanoEthics,* Vol. 2, pp. 317–27

Schoenbaum, S. C. (2001). The Impact of Pandemic Influenza, with Special Reference to 1918. *International Congress Series,* Vol. 1219, (October, 2001), pp. 43-51.

Sharma, D. (2007). Technogenesis Redesigns Phylogenesis: Or, When Liberation Biology Meets Our Posthuman Future. *Biotechnology Law Report,* Vol. 26, No. 6, (December, 2007), pp. 575-82, eISSN 0730-031X.

Sheetz, T., Vidal, J., Pearson, T. D., & Lozano, K. (2005). Nanotechnology: Awareness and Societal Concerns. *Technology in Society,* Vol. 27, No. 3, (August, 2005), pp. 329-45, eISSN 0160-791X.

Song, R. (2009). Genetic Manipulation and the Resurrection Body, In: *The Bioethics of Regenerative Medicine,* K.-T. Ip, pp. 27-45, Springer, 978-1-4020-8966-4, Netherlands

Steinbock, B. (2008). Designer Babies: Choosing Our Children's Genes. *The Lancet,* Vol. 372, No.9646, (October, 2008), pp. 1294-95, eISSN 1474-547X.

Stich, S. P. (1978). The Recombinant DNA Debate. Philosophy & Public Affairs, Vol. 7, pp. 187-205

Taniguchi, N. (1974). On the Basic Concept of 'Nano-Technology', Proceedings of the International Conference on Production Engineering, Part II, Tokyo, JSPE 2, pp.18-23, 1974.

Thomson, J. A., et al. (1998). Embryonic Stem Cell Lines Derived from Human Blastocysts. *Science,* Vol. 282, No. 5391, (November, 1998), pp. 1145-7, ISSN 0036-8075

van der Burg, W. (1991). The Slippery Slope Argument. *Ethics,* Vol. 102, No. 1, pp. 42-65 van Ommen, G. J., Bakker, E., & den Dunnen, J. T. (1999). The Human Genome Project and the Future of Diagnostics, Treatment, and Prevention. *Lancet,* Vol. 354, Suppl. 1, (July, 1999), pp. S5-10, ISSN 0140-6736.

Xia, T., Li, N., & Nel, A. E. (2009). Potential Health Impact of Nanoparticles. *Annual Review of Public Health,* Vol. 30, (April 2009), pp. 137-50, eISSN 1545-2093.